The Sound Hoof:
Horse Health From the Ground Up

Lisa Simons Lancaster

Foreword
Fran Jurga

TALLGRASS
PUBLISHERS,
LLC

Larkspur, Colorado

Book Design: Grant Dunmire
Attention Media Group
Denver, Colorado

Illustrations: Carla Stroh

Anatomical Drawings: Kara Nichole Corps

Cover Photograph: John Miller, www.spectrumphotography.net

Copyright ©2004 by Tallgrass Publishers, LLC. All rights reserved. Printed in the United States of America. No part of this book may be reproduced or transmitted in any form or by any means, electronic or mechanical, including photocopying, recording, internet, or by any information storage and retrieval system without written permission of the Publisher.

Library of Congress Cataloging-In-Publication Data
ISBN 0-9645982-7-2

1. Horses   2. Horse Hoof Care   3. Equine Health
4. Natural Hoof Care   5. Alternative Veterinary Medicine   6. Farriery

FIRST EDITION

Tallgrass Publishers, LLC. titles include:
Equine Acupressure: A Working Manual
The Well-Connected Dog: A Guide to Canine Acupressure
Acu-Cat: A Guide to Feline Acupressure
Meridian Charts for Horses, Dogs and Cats

Tallgrass Publishers' titles may be purchased for business, promotional use, or special sales. Contact: www.tallgrasspublishers.com   email: tallgrasspub@earthlink.net
4559 Red Rock Drive
Larkspur, CO 80118
888-841-7211

Information provided in *The Sound Hoof: Horse Health From the Ground Up* is not a substitute for responsible veterinary and farriery care. Please consult your professional equine healthcare providers.

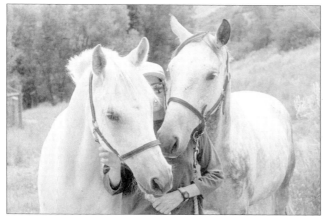

Eddie and Azulina

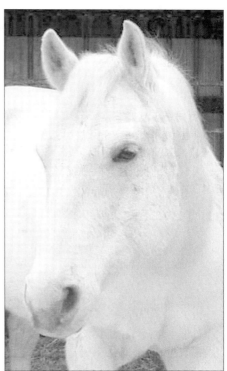

Mr. Skeeter

Dedication

To horses, with recognition of four who are most dear to my heart. Thanks to Oedipus, Azulina, Soupi, and Mr. Skeeter for the lessons you have taught me.

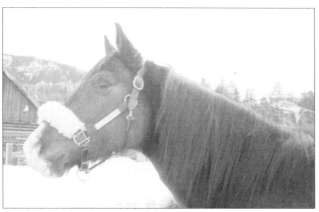

Soupi

Table of Contents

Foreword by Fran Jurga		vii
Introduction		xi
Chapter One	Holistic Hoof Care	1–6
	Holistic Practitioner	
	Chronic Condition Issue	
	The Farrier's Role in Holistic Hoof Care	
	Horseman's Role in Holistic Hoof Care	
Chapter Two	Hoof & Lower Leg Anatomy	7–20
	Terminology	
	Anatomical Structure	
Chapter Three	Reading the Hoof	21–44
	Evaluating Soundness	
	Understanding Balance	
	Three Dimensional Balance	
Chapter Four	Hoof Care Research & Theory	45–56
	The Nature of Research	
	Hoof Deformation Research	
	Brief History of Hoof Deformation Research	
	Breakover	
	Four-Point Trim and Natural Balance	
Chapter Five	To Shoe or Not to Shoe	57–71
	Balance	
	Contraction	
	Advantages of Barefoot	
	Disadvantages of Barefoot	
	Things to Discuss with Your Farrier	
	Dealing with Pain	
Chapter Six	Laminitis and Navicular	73–92
	Laminitis	

CHAPTER SIX   LAMINITIS AND NAVICULAR (CONTINUED)   73–92
    What is Laminitis
    Causes and Mechanisms of Laminitis
    Metabolically Based Theories
    How is Laminitis Diagnosed?
    How Do You know If Your Horse is Laminitic?
    What to do If You Suspect Laminitis
    Prevention and Treatment
    Navicular Syndrome
    Clinical Signs of Navicular
    Diagnosing Navicular
    Speculative Mechanisms and Risk Factors
    Relationship Between Inner and Outer Hoof Structures
    Prevention and Treatment of Heel Pain
    Foam Padding for Heel Pain
    A Holistic Approach

CHAPTER SEVEN   SOUND MANAGEMENT   93–100
    Support Team
    Selecting a Farrier
    How to Keep a Farrier
    Doing Your Own Trimming
    Safety
    Record keeping
    Scheduling
    Your Horse's Health is in Your Hands

CHAPTER EIGHT   ACTION GALLERY   101–111

SUMMARY   113
HOOF REPORT CARD   115
SELECTED RESOURCES   117
SELECTED REFERENCES   119
PHOTOGRAPHY & ART CREDITS   122
INDEX   123
ACKNOWLEDGEMENTS   124
ABOUT THE AUTHOR   125

Foreword

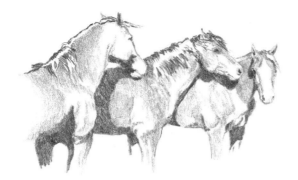

Not too many years ago, whenever I mentioned to horse owners that I was interested in hooves and wrote about them exclusively, I could be sure that conversation would halt. They didn't know what to say next. It was awkward.

Owners did not want to be reminded that their horses had feet. Four of them, no less. Four chances to go lame at every step. "How interesting," they would murmur evasively.

How things have changed. Now everyone wants to tell me about their horses' hooves, and they are full of questions: What do I think about hoof boots? And what about the barefoot trims? Do I know a good farrier? What about white line disease?

Overnight, it seems, there has been a surge in awareness of the importance of feet in horse health and soundness. Different hoof care regimen and shoeing styles are followed as religiously as diets and exercise programs for people.

How sound is your horse? Does "sound" mean merely "not lame" or is it a higher state of health and comfort? Would you feel the difference from the saddle if your horse's feet were less contracted, better balanced, free of cracks or thrush or whatever else you think is "wrong" with them? Would your horse's overall attitude, posture, and energy level improve if his feet were healthier?

If you answered, "I'm not sure" to these questions, congratulations. Chances are that you're being honest. And you're far from alone.

When shown a photo of a healthy foot, most owners--and many farriers, too--will assume that the foot must be attached to a wild horse from the American West, or a tough native breed known for robust feet. It looks healthy, but also strangely foreign. Feet like that aren't walking around the showground. You don't see them in the Futurity. They're not in the sales catalogues. And, they're certainly not in your barn. Or mine.

Most of us settle for "normal" feet functioning reasonably well so that the horse moves comfortably and freely, and so that we don't see any external signs of damage, distortion, or cracks.

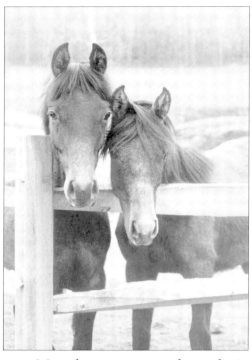
Lisa Lancaster wants to change that. She wants us not to ask more of our horses' feet, but to give them more. More care, more thought and more of a vision of how healthy and sound they could be one day.

Normal is just not good enough any more for Lisa and for a new legion of owners, farriers, and veterinarians who want to stretch the envelope of what we can do to help our horses achieve a higher level of long-term, maintainable balance and soundness.

Seeing the potential rather than the problems in a horse's feet is the place for us to begin. What should a horse's feet look like? What red flags are written in his medical history or his bloodlines? How limiting are his conformation challenges? Are we willing to stick with this horse for the long haul and help him stand on the best possible feet?

Many horse owners make apologies for being absentee owners. Most need to work outside the barn to pay for the barn. They buy horses raised and trained by others, hopefully more knowledgeable and skilled at choosing a stallion for a mare, at raising foals, at training young horses. They are riding the fruits of their labors, or paying the vet bills for the consequences of their mistakes.

In this book, Lisa Lancaster exhorts us to stop apologizing for not being the textbook-prescribed, hands-on owners of the last century. At the same time she urges us to take responsibility for our horses' soundness and to re-define the average owner's role as the primary caregiver, with the backup of a sympathetic, and synergistic professional support network.

The variables in our horses' lives seem designed to make hoof care a frustrating but necessary regimen. A horse may be bought and sold several times in its life, its environment is plagued by fluctuations between wet and dry, its feet may need to be cosmetically trimmed or polished for show appearance. It is trimmed and/or shod by farriers of different abilities and philosophies, its exercise is limited, and its basic nutrition is artificially supplemented with high-caloric grain products because good green healthy pasture time is becoming an ancestral memory for many of our equine friends.

If you make the commitment to work for and with your horse to improve his soundness, you will need to follow Lisa's advice and look for professionals who not only share your vision, but who know how to attain it.

Those people are hard to find, and you must earn their trust and support. Chances are they won't be in your backyard. You may have to haul your horse to a farrier, or fly across the country to attend a seminar with a specialist veterinarian. You will have to get your hands dirty, and your horse will have to learn to pick his feet up and stand still, at the same time, once and for all. And not just for you, but for anyone.

Most of all, you will have to learn to trust your horse, and he you. Following Lisa's program for holistic hoof health will be a lot of work, at first. Then it will become second nature, and soon you may find yourself staring at your horse's hoofprints in the sand of an arena and realizing that each one of them is telling you a story.

But, wait, look closer, there's more: You're in there too. You've made those hoofprints possible, by caring for and about your horse and his feet.

Learning how to look is what this book is about.

If you were shown the photos of ten horses' feet, could you pick out your horse's foot? After reading this book, I am sure that you will be able to do that.

But remember that Lisa is asking much, much more of you. She is asking you to go beyond mere awareness of and concern for your horse's feet. She is asking you to connect the dots between his hooves and the rest of his body, to see the connections between health, soundness, and sanity. She is asking you to visualize what his feet could look like if they were balanced and healthy, and how relaxed and content he could be for years to come if his feet were the strong foundation of his overall health equation.

– Fran Jurga
Hoofcare & Lameness
Journal of Equine
Foot Science
Gloucester,
Massachusetts
July 2004

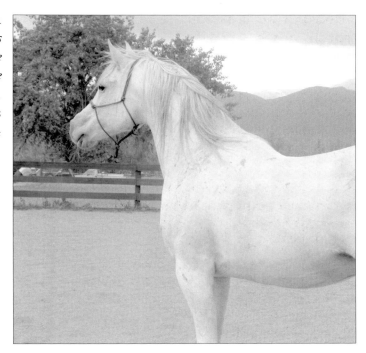

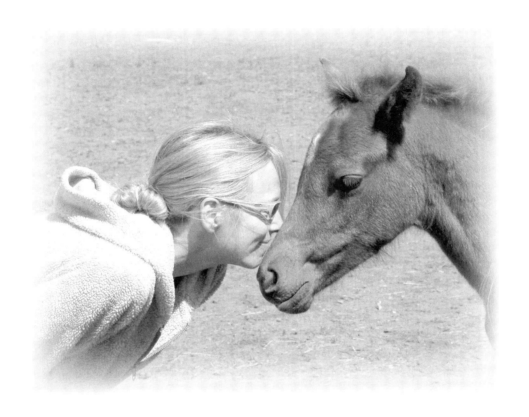

Wherever man has left his footprint in the long ascent to civilization we will find the hoofprint of the horse beside it.
— John Trotwood Moore

Introduction

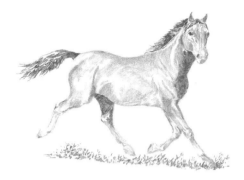

A perfectly balanced foot means perfect rest while standing and perfectly free and easy movements while in motion…
— David Roberge,
The Foot of the Horse, 1894

The sound of horse hooves evokes what every horseman feels about these awe-inspiring creatures. From the peaceful rhythm of a single horse walking on a hard surface to the thunder of a herd galloping, the cadence resonates within each of us. The beat of hooves captures the essence of the equine spirit: power, grace, and movement. In myth and in fact, the horse has thus been represented as a creature of flight and speed. Heads up, manes flowing, tails flying, horses seem to soar across any terrain: muddy, sandy, rocky, hard or soft. Their hooves have a remarkable combination of sensitivity and toughness. A horse can sense changes in ground surface in a fraction of a second, adjust hoof placement, and maintain a smooth, strong, efficient stride without missing a beat.

Inspired by the elegant and agile movement of the horse, farriers, veterinarians, and scientists have studied the design and function of the hoof and limb. The more we understand about the biological engineering of the horse's hoof, the better equipped we become to preserve soundness in these marvelous animals.

To achieve and maintain soundness is the goal of any hoof care plan. There are multiple approaches to attain this goal. It is no easy task for the horse owner to find the key to soundness for each horse. For every possible method of hoof care there is a different, sometimes totally opposite approach. What works on some horses does not work on all horses.

How is the horse owner to sort through the conflicting claims, research findings, and opinions of farriers, veterinarians, and researchers? The first step is for you to gather information. To that end, *The Sound Hoof* provides the reader with enough background and current hoof care theory to begin making informed choices. Additionally, the interested horse owner is encouraged to learn as much as possible about different methods of hoof care by attending clinics or reading the original works of different practitioners.

The Sound Hoof demystifies current trimming and shoeing practices rather than serving as a proponent for one particular theory or technique. In every-day language,

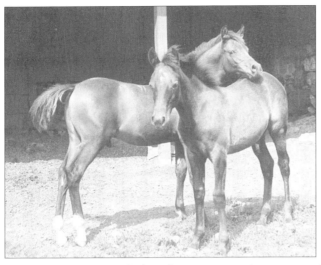 this book provides the reader with the principles underlying hoof care along with methods to evaluate competing claims. After reading *The Sound Hoof*, horse-care providers will have the essential tools with which to make their own educated decisions.

Regardless of the trimming or shoeing method you ultimately select, the central message of this book is that perpetual balance is a possibility for your horse. No two horses will respond exactly the same way to a specific hoof care protocol, yet every horse will achieve maximum benefit from having balanced feet all of the time.

A domesticated horse usually cannot maintain his own perfect balance. It is the owner's obligation to provide hoof care services. Everyone in hoof care will tell you that balance is important and is usually attainable, to a varying degree, each time the horse is seen by the farrier. What you will hear less often is the notion that perpetual balance is one secret to lifelong soundness and maximum performance.

Perfect perpetual balance, for numerous reasons, will not be attainable for every horse. But to strive for it will give every horse the best chance to move as efficiently as conformation and circumstance will allow. This book explains why most horses are not in perpetual balance and what you can do to improve the situation for your horse.

The Sound Hoof demystifies current trimming and shoeing practices.

The Sound Hoof will help readers answer the following questions:
- What does your horse need to be in perpetual balance?
- What is holistic hoof care?
- What are the main structures and functions of the hoof?
- What are the goals of shoeing and trimming?
- What are the main controversies among hoof studies today?
- Can you do your own trimming?
- How can you choose the right farrier for each horse?

- How can you help your horses if they have been diagnosed with navicular, laminitis, or other common hoof pathologies?
- What resources exist to help you learn more about holistic hoof and health care?

Veterinarians and farriers do not always know why a horse is lame, but everyone wants them to be sound. Symptomatic relief is the demand placed on hoof care practitioners. Horses, from pasture pets to pleasure mounts to world-class athletes, are often made temporarily sound only to come up lame again. Horse owners may resent veterinarians or farriers who suggest that the horse be given a long rest period, a whole season off, or turned out in the pasture barefoot. They often demand treatment for a lame horse in order to prolong its working life. Thus conventional hoof care practitioners tend to respond with the immediate goal of alleviating symptoms rather than finding a long-term solution to lameness.

Perpetual balance is one secret to lifelong soundness and maximum performance.

Nineteenth-century farrier David Roberge was an avid proponent of frequent hoof care. He reminded owners not to be too quick to cast blame on the shoe or trim method when a horse was lame, but rather to recognize and act upon the requirement to maintain perpetual balance. His words capture the core values of this book.

> Too many owners of horses…attribute to bad shoeing those results which ought to be laid to the account of neglecting to have the horses' feet pared down and shod regularly and sufficiently often … injuries caused by the overgrowth of the hoof even while the horse is standing still are much greater than hard work would be with feet kept to the natural size …
>
> A growing hoof is a growing evil, and the longer the space of time between each paring or trimming the foot, even supposing it to be done well, so will be the magnitude of the evil… The fault then, is in neglecting to pare the foot monthly or oftener if it needs it.
>
> Owners of horses cannot be impressed too deeply with the importance of this fact as one of the absolute requirements of the horse, the neglect of which are penalties of a very serious nature…
>
> Horses of every age and description or form or texture of feet, as long as they live, are amenable to treatment. I have had some cases that were **very aged** who, after their feet were expanded, would **hop, skip, and jump** like colts at play. Horses raised under the careful watching management and shod upon principles and practice I am endeavoring to inculcate, may be taken to market as perfect as the day they were foaled.

Everyone likes to see a horse "hop, skip, and jump like colts at play." What can you do to insure your horse the kind of joyful existence that comes from pain-free feet? As the caring owners of the horse, we are all responsible for providing the best for these incredible animals to maintain a lifetime of soundness and balance.

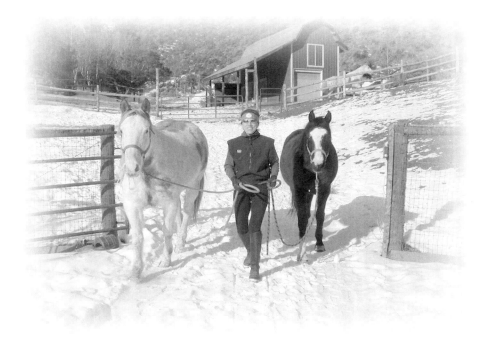

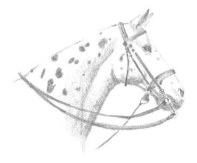

chapter one

Holistic Hoof Care

- **Goals of Holistic Hoof Care**
- **Holistic Farrier**
- **Chronic Conditions**
- **Holistic Farrier's Role**
- **Horse Owner's Role**

Nature has bestowed upon the horse an extraordinary foot: sensitive, resilient and sturdy. With their evolutionary imperative to take flight from danger, horses' hooves are designed for rapid and efficient movement. While the domestic horse is rarely required to run for the sake of survival, it is still the horses' genetic endowment to have strong, capable hooves. Horses' feet withstand a stunning array of forces as they run, slide, jump, spin and climb. What can you do to ensure that your horse's feet live up to their maximum potential for a lifetime of strength and resilience? The first step is a realization that a horse's hoof is not separate from the rest of its body. The health of the hoof is related to the health of the horse, and vice versa. You can provide care emphasizing the organic, functional relation between the parts and the entire equine body.

Holistic Hoof Care

This book is an expression of the holistic belief that good hoof care is necessary but by itself is not enough for optimal hoof health. Optimal health requires overall holistic management principles. Holistic hoof care means that the whole horse must be balanced in order to achieve the strongest possible feet.

Because the word holistic is usually associated with medicine, it is important to clarify the role of the farrier as distinct from, yet complementary to, the role of the veterinarian. The farrier, like the chiropractor or acupressurist, does not diagnose or treat disease. The chiropractor aligns the spine; the acupressurist balances the energy; and the farrier aligns the hoof and lower leg.

Posture and normal physiology are interrelated: how the horse's hoof is balanced and how the horse lands and loads each foot affects the physiological function of many body systems, most significantly the nervous and musculoskeletal

Holistic hoof care means that the whole horse must be balanced in order to achieve the strongest possible feet.

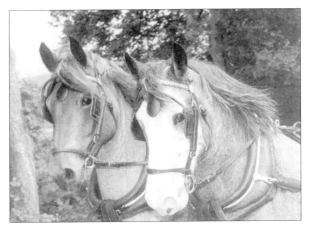

systems. If problems are alleviated by chiropractic or farrier care, it is through balance that the healing power of the body has been restored.

Holistic approaches to health are centered on the concept of homeostasis. That is, the body's ability to maintain stable internal conditions in the face of changing external conditions. Homeostasis is dynamic equilibrium. Internal conditions change within narrow limits. Metabolism is in balance when all body systems, including the hooves, are operating properly. Imbalance anywhere, if not corrected quickly, is likely to result in compensatory imbalance somewhere else.

The delicate balance of homeostasis is more easily maintained than restored. Holistic hoof care excels at maintaining "hoof homeostasis." Holistic care can also assist in the re-establishment of homeostasis, but the primary goal is the achievement of perpetual balance.

The goal of a holistic hoof care approach first and foremost is to prevent disease or discomfort. This approach can also offer options differing from conventional approaches for treating common hoof dysfunctions. Like the distinction between a holistic medical practitioner and a conventional medical practitioner, a holistic farrier differs from a conventional farrier.

Holistic Practitioner

In choosing a holistic practitioner, whether farrier or veterinarian, you can make the best health care choices when you have a clear understanding of the difference between holistic and conventional. People associate holistic practice with nutritional, herbal, or homeopathic treatments and conventional practice with drugs and surgery. This division of "modalities" is only a partial distinction between approaches and will not always help you to make informed choices.

In the words of holistic veterinarian Russell Swift, "It is not the procedure or substance that determines whether something is holistic or not. It is the philosophy behind the method that counts. Any of the so-called 'holistic' therapies can be used in 'conventional' way." For example, using acupressure or acupuncture instead of injecting drugs into sore hock joints may appear holistic. But unless the underlying cause of the sore hock is addressed, the treatment, being only symptomatic, is unlikely to result in complete healing.

Dr. Swift defines the holistic practitioner as one who sees holistic health as a commitment, not a commodity. Currently, "holistic" is a common buzzword that brings in more business. Swift warns consumers to beware of practitioners with limited holistic training. They may have fancy advertising in the yellow pages and claim to "prefer" using natural remedies, but in practice they prescribe the usual round of drugs, such as cortisone or antibiotics for health problems that may have been amenable to less invasive and less extreme methods.

The holistic practitioner is concerned not only with the least invasive methods of care, but with assessing the bigger picture. This bigger picture for the horse includes the relationship between horse and owner. The holistic farrier is not just "shoeing feet." A holistic farrier considers the expectation for the horse's level of performance along with the owner's needs. A horse may not need shoes; but if the owner cannot provide appropriate barefoot hoof care and protection, the holistic farrier balances needs and provides appropriate service for the horse in relation to the owner's requirements.

The holistic practitioner understands that the whole horse cannot be properly assessed independently from its caregiver. This is an essential yet often overlooked point. A farrier does not shoe every horse as if it were his very own.

In the real world, horses, working with their owners, perform jobs far beyond what nature demands. The holistic farrier will be able to inform the owner if there is a potential conflict between the shoeing a horse needs for soundness and the work the animal is expected to perform. There are times when a farrier could provide shoeing that would permit the horse to keep working but may impair the foot's own capacity to heal or stay healthy. At that point, the horse owner, with the farrier's guidance, must make the best decision given his or her priorities in relation to the health and welfare of the horse.

Because it is not technique alone that defines holistic practice, the mark of a qualified and experienced holistic farrier is being able to assess each case individually to determine the need for different shoeing or trimming options. The holistic farrier is knowledgeable regarding barefoot hoof care, but not by definition limited to it. The needs of the horse/owner team take priority over any one type of hoof care. This is the defining spirit of holistic health – accounting for and balancing the needs of the whole animal in the context of the human-animal bond.

The same principles apply to the holistic veterinarian. The capable and experienced practitioner will know when to use drugs or surgery versus when less invasive methods might work. Does your veterinarian see holistic health as a commodity or a commitment?

> **The holistic practitioner understands that the whole horse cannot be properly assessed independently from its caregiver.**

The "commodity" perspective sounds like this: when normal medical approaches to disease have been exhausted and the patient no longer responds, then alternative approaches probably will do no harm and may make the horse owner feel better. In contrast, a committed holistic practitioner would try the least invasive and less extreme methods first and go on to other resources as needed given the animal's condition.

Chronic Condition Issue

The challenge, particularly with chronic conditions, is to determine which conditions are incurable. In conventional hoof care, for example, many problems are considered incurable, and palliative measures are considered the best possible approach. A holistic perspective takes a case-by-case approach. Holistic farriers often find that some of these "incurable" horses, for example those diagnosed with navicular, ringbone, or severe laminitis, can become sound and return to performing at high levels.

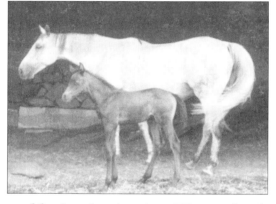

If you have been around horses for a while you have heard the term "serviceably sound." It expresses our awareness that a horse is not entirely comfortable but is nonetheless able to work for us despite some degree of pain.

A serviceably sound horse is not normally the subject of extensive veterinary investigation but rather is one shod in whatever manner seems to arrest visible signs of further deterioration. We say of such horses there is a "hitch in their get-a-long", "this is just how they are," or it's their "way of going." If nothing we've tried has improved the horse's comfort, we simply endeavor to keep things from getting worse.

Is this the best that can be expected? Should you resign your horse to a life of being so-called, "serviceably sound?" There are no simple answers. Yet holistic hoof care suggests there is more room for improvement than many people have been led to believe.

The Farrier's Role in Holistic Hoof Care

The farrier's job is to keep the horse's feet maintained so the animal is comfortable and the entire body is dynamically balanced. Just like our hair and nails, horses' feet grow constantly. Unless your horse is barefoot and gets enough exercise to keep the feet worn down, hoof wall will grow forward and away from the center of balance of the horse's leg, in which case, someone must nip or rasp off the excess growth. Usually, the longer the hoof has grown between trim or shoe appointments, the more out of balance the horse will be.

On a six-to-eight-week schedule, a farrier can only re-establish balance with each visit. The holistic approach is focused on prevention rather than reaction to problems. Since maintaining balance is the priority for the holistic farrier, he or she will recommend frequent appointments to keep the foot under the horse, thus preserving consistent balance.

Horse owners expect to see their horses' feet look neat and nicely shaped right after the farrier has worked on the foot. People have become accustomed to watching a horse's feet slowly get long, unbalanced, flared, cracked, or otherwise distorted enough to look as if they are ready for the farrier's next visit. An important principle explained in this book is that if feet look overgrown to the untrained eye, they probably have been out of balance for far too long.

Controversy flares around the definition of normal. Normal is usually defined by whatever keeps that horse sound. Yet many horses will be sound for a while and then become lame; in which case the "normal" way the foot was being trimmed or shod might not have been optimal for that horse.

If placed in an ideal environment, the horse would maintain its own feet. Rate of wear would equal rate of growth. When the hoof horn is covered with a shoe, we completely eliminate the possibility of the hooves wearing at all. Even if our domesticated horses remain barefoot, it takes a lot of riding to keep their feet from needing a trim.

If the horse is shod, how do you know what kind of shoeing or trimming is best, and what intervals are best for your horses? We can safely say that maintaining balance is an important measure to prevent lameness. Balance cannot be perfectly maintained in the shod horse but can be approximated within reasonable limits if shod frequently enough. If farrier appointments are far apart, the feet will be out of balance for more of the time than they are in balance. Horses manage to adapt to being out of balance. People are accustomed to seeing feet that are "due for new shoes." However, the time spent out of balance may impact the longer term health of the hoof and the horse.

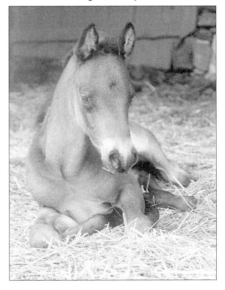

The key to hoof health is to keep the hoof within the narrow limits of balance. Slightly too short, too long, or off-balance is never ideal, but the horse can cope temporarily. Chronically short, long or unbalanced feet will eventually cause dysfunction and, if left long enough, irreversible degeneration.

Appointments with a holistic farrier are usually more frequent, and often take longer for each visit. The length of the visit is determined in part by the need for the farrier to take a detailed history and keep extensive records for each visit. Signs that might be insignificant to a conventional farrier or veterinarian take on significance to a holistic practitioner. Every bump, scratch, and hoof horn deviation will be noted in the horse's chart.

The horse's personality and emotional response to different shoes, and to the shoeing appointment itself are important. For example, your holistic farrier will take a history that includes all the types of shoeing that have been tried in the past and how your horse responded to each. Any sign of discomfort during the actual shoeing process will be noted. For instance, some horses are uncomfortable holding their legs for the farrier. Some are uncomfortable when nails are struck. Not everything will be meaningful, but unless it is all written down, it will be forgotten, and potentially important clues and patterns over time will be missed.

A holistic farrier will work with the owner to establish a comprehensive hoof care plan to meet the needs of both horse and rider. This is much like a personal trainer who helps you at the gym but also addresses lifestyle issues, such as health and nutrition history and habits.

Holistic farriers work within a network of veterinarians, chiropractors, acupressurists, bodyworkers, and other equine health professionals. For example, if your farrier notices mild signs of hoof distortion in a previously sound horse, rather than taking a wait-and-see approach, your farrier might refer you to an equine chiropractor who can assess a possible locomotion or skeletal problem.

Maintaining soundness requires vigilance. The goal is to prevent tiny signs from becoming overt lameness. The chiropractor, in turn, may find that spinal manipulation will help the horse but that other modalities such as massage, acupressure, or physical therapy, are needed to restore proper musculoskeletal function.

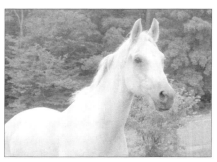

Horseman's Role in Holistic Hoof Care

Ultimately, it is the horse owner who is responsible for the horse's hoof care. This does not mean, however, the owner does all of the direct care. Horse owners who have taken an active role in their horse's hoof health have found value in a team approach. The two main pillars of the team will always be you and your farrier. Some horse owners seek specific training and then perform their own routine hoof care, calling in the farrier intermittently for special circumstances. Others prefer to hire a professional farrier to do the work, but these owners maintain an active role in hoof care decision-making.

chapter two

Hoof and Lower Leg Anatomy

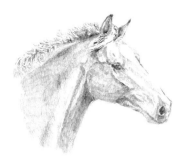

- **Anatomical Reference Terminology**
- **Bone Structure**
- **Hoof Structure and Research**

Throughout history, nature's intricate design for the hoof has driven farriers, veterinarians, and researchers to study and write about its anatomy and physiology. A properly functioning hoof is the foundation of equine magnificence. The splendor of a healthy horse playfully engaging in acrobatic antics with a pasture-mate, the power of a racehorse pounding down the homestretch, the grace of a sport horse performing lightening-fast reining patterns: to engage fully in these activities, a horse needs to be sound. We owe our horses a lifetime of pain-free, perfectly functioning feet. Knowing how the hoof works and the remarkable role that it plays in keeping your horse sound is key in determining how and when his hooves should be trimmed and shod.

This chapter will help you visualize the significant anatomical structures of the horse's foot. As you learn the anatomy and some basic physiology you will see how the exterior indicators of hoof health relate to the internal alignment of bones and soft tissues. Additionally, you will understand how the breakdown of this natural function can cause your horse pain and lameness. The more you know about these issues, the better equipped you will be to facilitate the important decisions regarding your horse's soundness. Although tendons and ligaments are important to the function of the hoof, discussion of these structures is beyond the scope of this book.

Terminology

In order to follow the anatomical descriptions you need to be familiar with some of the common navigational terms. There are many planes of reference describing anatomical directions and locations. Imagine that you are on the phone with your veterinarian or farrier, and want to describe something you see on your horse's hoof or pastern. The person on the phone is not able to see what you see. You must use a shared language of anatomical reference points so that the person with whom you are talking can visualize the location you describe. Some of the terms used in the veterinary and farrier world are: proximal, distal, dorsal, palmar, caudal, solar, lateral, medial, anterior, and posterior.

Proximal and Distal

Proximal means toward the body; that is, the proximal pastern bone is the long pastern bone since it is the closest foot bone to the body. Distal means away from the body; that is, the distal foot bone is the coffin bone since it is the furthest bone away from the horse's body. Proximal and distal are terms used to describe a limb bone in relation to other limb bones, or a part of a bone in relation to the rest of the bone. For example, the distal tip of the coffin bone is the furthest point from the body, the tip of the bone near the sole. The proximal portion of the coffin bone is the upper portion, the part including the extensor process.

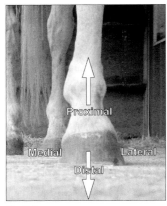

Fig 2.1a

Solar, Palmar, Caudal, Dorsal

Solar refers to the ground surface of the foot, the sole. Palmar means the part of the foot or leg toward the rear of the horse. The portion of the foot toward the back is also referred to as the caudal area of the hoof. The expression "palmar foot pain," or "caudal foot pain" is often used to describe problems in the navicular area. In this case, palmar is used interchangeably with caudal, meaning the area of the foot around the heels. Dorsal means towards the spine or top of the animal, (like a dorsal fin on a dolphin), and ventral means down toward the abdominal mid-line. In relation to the hoof, dorsal refers to the front surface of the hoof wall or coffin bone, and ventral means towards the sole or ground.

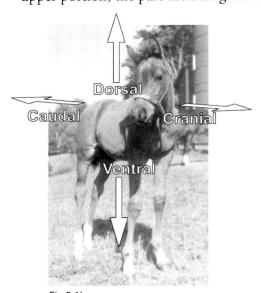

Fig 2.1b

Medial and Lateral/Dorsal and Palmar

The lateral side of the foot is the outer side; it is the view you have when standing on the left side of the horse looking at the left foot. The medial side of the foot or leg is the inside, closest to the horse's centerline. When standing on the left side of the horse, the medial side of the right leg can be seen, it is the side that has the chestnut. Dorsal means the view when you are standing in front of the horse

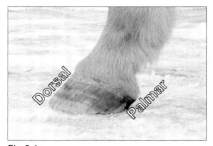

Fig 2.1c

facing the horse's head. Palmar means the view you have when standing directly behind the horse looking at the tail and toward the head. Often the term anterior (cranial) is used instead of dorsal, and posterior (caudal) used interchangably with palmar, strictly speaking, only the terms dorsal and palmar refer to the hoof.

Anatomical Structure

Coffin Bone

There are three bones in the horse's hoof. The most distal of these bones is commonly called the coffin bone. In the scientific literature the coffin bone is known as the third phalanx (P3), the pedal bone, or the distal phalanx. In most domestic horses the coffin bone lies entirely within the hoof capsule. Occasionally the proximal portion of the coffin bone, called the extensor process, is just above the hoof capsule at the coronet.

The coffin bone is an irregular shape with a complex three-dimensional form. In order to understand the form and function of this bone it helps to be able to visualize its various bony extensions and to see anatomical specimens cut along different planes. This will also help you appreciate x-ray views of the foot. The extensor process, sometimes called the pyramidal process, is the proximal tip of the dorsal surface of the bone. This is where the extensor tendon is attached. The normal position for the coffin bone is high enough within the hoof capsule for the extensor process to be almost at the level of the coronet. In foundered horses when the coffin bone sinks and/or rotates, the extensor process becomes markedly distal to the coronary band. This is visible

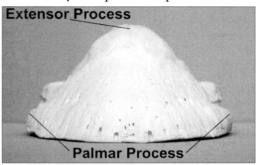
Fig 2.2a Front (anterior view) of the coffin bone shows entire dorsal surface.

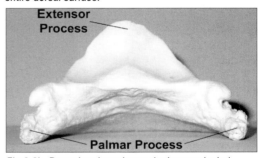
Fig 2.2b Posterior view shows the bottom (solar) surface and joint surfaces.

on x-rays and can be detected without x-rays in some cases when there is a pronounced dip or when you can push your finger into the top of the hairline.

The front surface of the coffin bone is called the dorsal surface. The bottom of the coffin bone is called the solar surface and the edge running around the bottom of the bone is called the distal border. The caudal part of the bone includes the palmar processes. Process means "bony prominence." Palmar processes are also called the "wings" of the coffin bone. The dorsal surface and extensor process are present at birth, but the palmar processes are not. The palmar processes develop slowly over the first few years of the horse's life. They are sometimes fractured in animals worked beyond their physical capacity. Because the palmar processes are less dense than the other parts of the coffin bone they are less noticeable on x-rays.

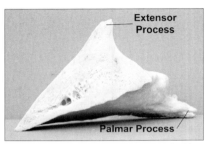

Fig 2.2c Sagittal cut section shows inside the coffin bone.

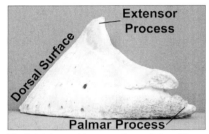

Fig 2.2d Lateral image of an adult coffin bone view shows palmar process.

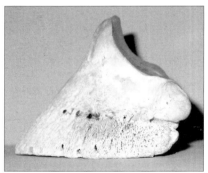

Fig 2.2e Lateral view of foal coffin bone, note that it does not have palmar processes.

The solar surface of the coffin bone is slightly concave or cupped. This concavity is mirrored in the vaulted surface of the sole that is noticeable when you look at your horse's feet. You may have noticed that hind feet tend to have a deeper concavity than the front feet. This is also reflected in the bones. Most front coffin bones are slightly less vaulted than hinds. The concavity of this half-moon shaped bone is not easily appreciated in certain cut sections or in x-ray views. One way hoof specimens are typically cut is in a sagittal section, cut vertically down the mid-line. To understand this plane, you must first recognize the median plane. The median plane divides the body or limb into two equal halves by slicing down the mid-line. A sagittal plane is a section cut parallel to the median plane. Sometimes the term "mid-sagittal" is used interchangeably with median.

Imagine a lower limb specimen cut into two equal halves. When looking at the cut edge of the foot in this sagittal view, the coffin bone looks like a triangular wedge. You see what looks like a sharp distal tip pointing towards the sole and the palmar processes are not visible in this view. When people first see this view of the foot bones, they often think the coffin bone looks rotated because the distal tip seems to be pointing down. An x-ray image appears similar to the sagittal view because the palmar processes, being a smaller area of bone, appear faint. Keep in mind the three-dimensional shape of the coffin bone and you will be able to appreciate the outline of the whole bone in an x-ray, or imagine the rest of it when you look at a sagittal section.

Navicular Bone

There is another important bone contained within the hoof capsule called the navicular bone. The navicular bone, sometimes called the distal sesamoid, also called nut bone or shuttle bone in older texts, is positioned at the back of the coffin bone above the attachment point of the deep flexor tendon. It appears to be designed to not bear weight directly. Sesamoid bones exist where tendons change direction. The horse has sesamoid bones at the fetlock, which are called proximal sesamoids. In the hoof, the distal sesamoid is the navicular bone.

The navicular bone, like the coffin bone, has an unusual three-dimensional form, which looks different depending on the angle from which it is seen. This small bone has a complex anatomy because it has one joint surface that contacts the coffin bone and another joint surface that contacts the distal end of the short pastern bone. It has yet another important surface that contacts the deep digital flexor tendon.

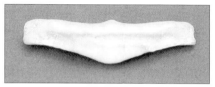

Fig 2.3 Navicular bone.

Navicular syndrome may be due to damage in the navicular bone, navicular bursa, surrounding tissues, or even in other parts of the foot. New anatomical findings about the soft tissues surrounding the navicular bone may offer clues about "caudal hoof pain". Currently, navicular disease syndrome is a prevalent problem in the equine population for which neither conclusive early detection nor successful treatment has been documented. (See Chapter 6 for discussion of navicular syndrome.)

Pastern Bones

The short pastern bone, also called the second phalanx, middle phalanx, or simply, P2, sits above of the coffin bone. About half of the bone is within the hoof capsule, half above it. When you push your fingers against your horse's leg at the coronary band, you are pressing the short pastern bone. Above the short pastern bone is the long pastern bone, known as P1, the first phalanx, or the proximal phalanx. This is the main bone of the fetlock. If you place your hand around the horse's fetlock, you are holding the long pastern bone.

The sesamoid bones, also called the proximal sesamoids, are located above P1. There are two sesamoid bones, one on each side of the back of the joint between P1 and the cannon bone.

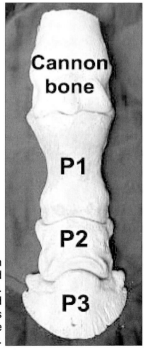

Fig 2.4a Pastern bones viewed from the front. Navicular and sesamoid bones are not visible from this view.

Metacarpal Bone

The cannon bone, also called the second metacarpal, is the main bone between the fetlock and the knee. The splint bones are tiny shafts of bone, one on either side of the cannon bone, which many people learn about when their horse is said to have "popped a splint." The splint bones are also called the first and third metacarpals.

Hoof Wall

The outer wall is the hard outer covering that is most easily recognizable, even to non-horse people, as the horse's hoof. The wall is somewhat analogous to our fingernail. It is "dead" tissue in that it has no blood or nerve supply and is made primarily of hardened protein tissue called keratin. Above the coronary band is the periolic ring. This is a band of soft tissue that produces the periople, a thin layer of skin that covers and protects the coronary band, in a gasket-like effect similar to the cuticle on your fingernail. The periople may be colorless or it may be white. It soaks up water, swells and becomes easier to see when the foot is wet.

The outer wall grows from the top down towards the ground. This is why you will often see a crack, bruise, or other defect growing down the hoof wall long after an injury occurred at the top. This is just like when you bruise your finger or toe and see the black mark grow out for weeks or months afterwards. Damaged wall cannot heal at the site of damage, but must grow out and be replaced by new horn.

The wall has long been considered the main weight bearing structure; but new research documents that the foot is designed to use the sole and frog in combination with the wall for ideal weight bearing. In some horses, when the wall has grown out to where the sole, bars and frog no longer touch the ground and serve as part of the weight bearing surface, the wall cannot withstand long-term stress.

Recent research has tested some of the basic claims about hoof wall loading patterns. Interestingly, scientific testing has overturned some of the strongly held beliefs about the ways in which the hoof is designed to contact the ground and to bear weight. See Chapter 4 for discussion of hoof wall loading and implications for trimming and shoeing.

Bars

The bars are a continuation of the wall. The bars seem to grow at the same rate as the wall but do not wear down as quickly because they are not in contact with the ground throughout their entire length.

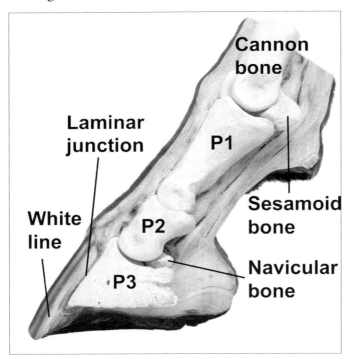

Fig 2.5 Lateral view of lower leg anatomy.

Bars, in the old farrier texts, were referred to as "braces." This is perhaps a more descriptive term capturing one of their known functions. The bars appear to act as springs to hold the back of the foot together, allowing it to move and keeping it from becoming too open which would flatten the foot, or too closed, which would contract the foot inwards.

Sole

Sole is a modified form of hard skin that covers the bottom of the horse's foot, and like the wall, the outer layer of the sole is not supplied with blood or nerves. The sole provides a protective covering for the sensitive structures and tissue beneath. The solar surface of the equine foot is slightly arched, following the contour of the bottom of the coffin bone.

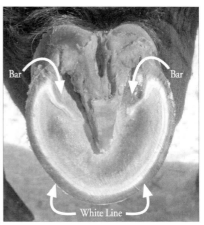

Fig 2.6 The bars are a continuation of the hoof wall as it bends around at the heel. The white line includes the bars.

Sole horn is softer than wall horn, but harder than frog horn. Trauma to the sole can cause bruising. The trauma may come from the environment, such as rocky terrain. Trauma can also occur from the inside of the foot causing bruising to appear externally on the sole, when the coffin bone presses against the sole in a foundered horse. In either case, the sole horn, like the wall horn when bruised, will contain evidence of trauma long after the insult has occurred. This is because horn tissue, unlike living tissue, has no blood supply of its own. Horn cannot heal from the outside in. Old bruises must grow out as new healthy horn grows from the inside and pushes bruised horn out.

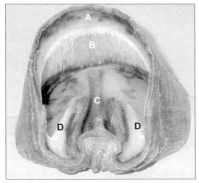

Fig 2.7 Empty hoof capsule, soft tissues removed. Inner structures include (A) coronary groove, (B) epidermal laminar horn of inner hoof wall, (C) frog, (D) bars. Note that bars are laminated like inner hoof wall.

There is not much research on the sole, but farrier Gene Ovnicek's use of the concept of "sole plane" has proven extremely helpful to farriers. The concept itself is not actually new, as farriers have for centuries talked about the trim line as the junction between wall and sole, describing the "live" sole as the un-exfoliated portion. Ovnicek has popularized the term in his teaching system of trimming and shoeing for natural balance.

Many farriers have used the sole plane-based guidelines to prepare the foot successfully. But locating the sole plane is by no means obvious to the inexperienced eye. Soles can develop any number of confounding characteristics that render the simple notion of sole plane difficult to identify. Sole may be too thin but still appear exfoliating, too thick but appear waxy and "live".

White Line

The white line is the junction between the wall and the sole. You see the white line when you look closely at the solar surface of the foot. It is actually more of a yellow color and is not really a line but more of a zone. When looking at the white line closely it looks like a series of tiny filaments similar to the underside of a mushroom. In healthy feet, the while line is a narrow band, usually less than 1/8 of an inch wide, all around the perimeter of the hoof and curving around along the bars at the heel.

The condition of the white line can be an indication of what the German anatomists term "the suspensory apparatus of the foot." The white line connects the wall and sole. Because these structures move slightly as the foot expands and contracts, the white line can indicate how much natural suspension and elasticity is in the foot. In shod feet the white line is not visible because the shoe is placed directly over the perimeter of the foot. Farriers inspect this area carefully when re-shoeing because it can give important clues regarding the health of the foot. If your horse is barefoot, you can inspect the white line every time you pick up the foot.

If the white line is stretched, as you commonly see in laminitic feet, filled with blood, or cracked open and separated, these can be indications of a damaged foot. The white line connects the sole with the wall below the coffin bone; it is a continuation of the laminae along the length of the coffin bone. When the white line is visibly damaged at the solar surface, it is possible that the laminae higher up in the hoof are also damaged. Sometimes you see what looks like a danger sign such as a cracked or elongated white line. This may simply be because the feet are overgrown. After being trimmed and balanced, a once messy white line may become perfectly normal. If the white line looks damaged even after the foot has been trimmed, your horse might need to be checked by a veterinarian.

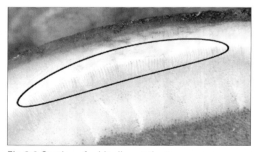

Fig 2.8 Section of white line at the toe.

When you look at the white line, you get an indication at the ground surface of what is happening to laminae higher in the hoof. You must clean off the foot and look very closely, but you can see with the unaided eye just how closely spaced the laminae are. If you take a photograph using a macro lens on a digital camera, and then look at this on your computer screen, you will get a very interesting view of your horse's white line. This would be a valuable image to keep in your horse's hoof health records file. You can compare changes over time, particularly if your horse is undergoing rehabilitation and needs to recover from past hoof distortion.

Laminae

The laminae, called lamellae by British and Australian hoof researchers, attach the coffin bone to the hoof wall. There are two interconnected layers, commonly called dermal and epidermal laminae that work together to keep the coffin bone in its normal position. The two layers fit together in a Velcro-like fashion.

The epidermal layer lines the inside of the hoof capsule and can be seen on the inner hoof wall in a specimen of an empty hoof capsule. The dermal layer wraps around the coffin bone and the rest of the inner foot and can be seen covering the bone on a specimen freshly separated from its hoof capsule. The dermal layer houses the blood and nerve supply of the hoof, while the epidermal layer is composed of horn and has no blood supply or nerves.

> ...scientific testing has documented that the true weight-bearing surface of the hoof includes parts of the sole, the frog, and the hoof wall.

Researchers have investigated the spacing and orientation of the laminae. Studies have shown that laminae are closer together at the toe than in the quarters. The laminae in the toe are aligned perpendicular to the wall at the toe, and are at an oblique angle in the quarters. Difference in laminar orientation may relate to different forces at the toe, quarter and heel.

Research by Robert Bowker, VMD, PhD, on laminar spacing suggests that laminar density is one mechanism by which the hoof may adapt to changing conditions. Research suggests that a hoof may adapt to changes in stress by altering the laminar density of the hoof. The laminar density can change depending on different forces on the hoof. For example, racehorse feet shod with toe grabs have higher density at the toe than feet without toe grabs. Laminar density has also been found to be higher on the flared side of an asymmetrical foot. These interesting findings show that the foot is highly adaptable, and can change quickly in response to different trimming and shoeing methods.

For centuries people have assumed that the hoof wall and laminae were the only support the bones in the hoof had. This belief was based on the fact that horses can perform when shod in an open shoe that provides support only around the perimeter of the foot. But just because the foot is able to function this way does not mean it is ideally designed to do so. Recent scientific

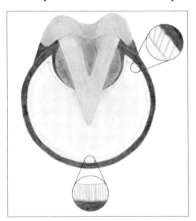

Fig 2.9 Illustration depicts white line laminae close together and perpendicular to hoof wall at the toe. In the heel area, the laminae are spaced further apart and their attachment between wall and sole is at an angle.

testing has documented that the true weight-bearing surface of the hoof includes parts of the sole, the frog, and the hoof wall. Studies of wild horse feet have shown that healthy hooves bear weight across much of the sole, frog, and even the heel bulbs. Research on domestic horses shows that on the natural deformable ground surface of a pasture, domestic barefoot horses also use more than just their hoof walls to hold their weight.

A common treatment of damaged horn wall involves removing part of the wall. The veterinarian will cut away the diseased horn or the farrier will "float" the ground surface so part of it is not touching the shoe. The horse will then walk on less than the whole wall. The rest of the foot adequately compensates for a temporary reduction of the ideal bearing surface. The main message is simply that multiple parts of the foot share the load. Compensation is a natural emergency "stop-gap" response. But over the long term, compensatory adaptation does not serve the horse well and future breakdown is likely.

Frog

The frog, located between the bars, like the wall and sole has a tough outer layer of horn tissue that protects the sensitive layer underneath. The frog contains the highest moisture content of all the outer hoof structures and is thus the most pliable.

The function of the frog has not been definitively determined, but it seems to act partly for traction and support. Also important in hoof physiology is the sensory function, which appears to be related to how the hoof interacts with the ground. Researcher Dr. Robert Bowker has documented the existence of pressure receptors in the frog. Without the base of the frog on the ground, the foot has reduced ability to feel the ground and to send messages from foot to brain. Be careful when interpreting this finding and applying it to how a horse should be trimmed. Lowering the heels so that the frog is bearing weight may or may not be called for in your horse's case. Realize that if a horse works on soft ground, the foot will sink in slightly and the frog will touch the ground, even if it would not touch the ground on a hard surface.

If left untrimmed too long, bar horn will grow over sole horn, and sometimes push against the frog, causing pressure and eventually bruising. In the healthy and well-proportioned foot, the bar, sole, frog and wall each occupy specific spaces, with none infringing upon the others. In neglected and off balance feet, bar can overgrow to cover much of the solar surface; frog can overgrow or it can shrink; sole can become too thick, referred to as false or retained sole.

There has been almost no research regarding the function of the frog, but practitioners see it as an important indicator of hoof health. Frogs that are an abnormal size, either too large or too small, or frogs that get recurrent infections such as thrush are indicators of hoof disease, imbalance, or both. Like the hoof wall and sole, the frog seems to be part of the support structure of the foot.

Lateral Cartilage

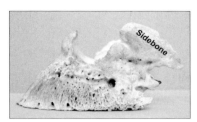

Fig 2.10 This specimen shows ossified lateral cartilage. Compare to other coffin bones shown in this chapter.

The hoof has two lateral cartilages in the back of the foot, one attached to each side of the coffin bone at the palmar processes. Ligaments hold the cartilage in place. The cartilage is located partly within the hoof capsule and partly above it. The top of the lateral cartilage can be felt just above the hairline at the back half of the foot. When you touch around the coronary band area at the back of the foot, you can feel the cartilage on both sides. In some horses the cartilage can ossify (turn to bone). This may be a sign that the feet have been off-balance for some time, or that the horse has been worked too hard and the foot was not able to effectively dissipate the shock.

Dr. Bowker's research shows that sound horses have thicker lateral cartilage and more blood vessels throughout this tissue than is present in horses with navicular lameness. In well-adapted feet, it seems that thicker, stronger cartilage combined with more vascular channels may offer efficient pressure regulation as blood flows through the vessels.

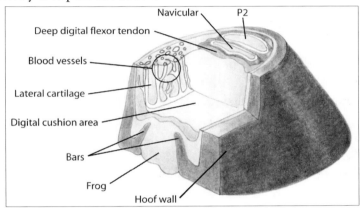

Fig 2.11 This drawing highlights the important anatomical fact that there are no bones in the back half of the hoof. The digital cushion is not drawn in this illustration. The large area between the lateral cartilages is where the digital cushion sits.

Digital Cushion

The digital cushion, also called the plantar cushion or distal cushion, is a mass of connective tissue located within the caudal hoof capsule. The digital cushion lies proximal to the frog and takes up most of the space in the back part of the foot between the lateral cartilages. The digital cushion has long been thought to play a role in shock absorption, but only recently has there been research that supports this idea. In addition, there is now scientifically documented detail about the structure and function of this important part of the foot. Dr. Bowker's research found that in pleasure horses euthanized due to navicular lameness, the digital cushion was a less supportive type of connective tissue than in sound horses euthanized for reasons other than lameness.

The digital cushion may be associated with pressure changes and blood flow within the palmar portion of the foot. Chapter 6 explores this topic in more detail.

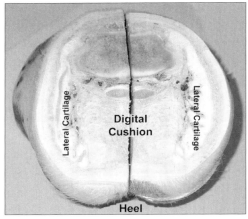

Fig 2.12 This specimen is cut in cross section at the level of the coronet. The digital cushion takes up the bulk of space across the middle of the foot and the lateral cartilages are on either side.

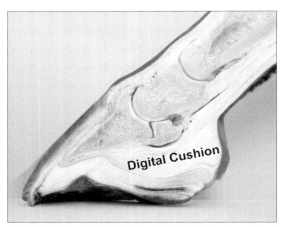

Fig 2.13 Sagittal view showing the digital cushion.

Summary

Knowledge of anatomy can help you identify warning signs in your horse's hoof. When you inspect the hoof carefully, what do you see in the white line? Is the sole concave, flat, or bulging outward? Can you feel hard lumps just above the hairline where the lateral cartilages emerge out of the hoof capsule?

Hoof capsule deviations suggest that the corresponding inner structures have lost their healthy form. A flat sole might mean the coffin bone is pressing down and resting too low in the hoof. A dished toe suggests that the laminae are not able to hold the coffin bone securely against the wall and the wall horn has consequently become distorted. A stretched white line is additional evidence that the coffin bone is not well suspended in the hoof capsule. You would need x-rays to confirm the position of the bone.

Not every deviation on the exterior form corresponds to an interior hoof problem. There are many possible causes of any single hoof form deviation. Yet once you know something about the relationship between structure and function, you are more likely to catch potential problems before they cause serious damage to your horse's feet.

With the knowledge from this chapter, you have enhanced your ability to communicate with your veterinarian and farrier. As you continue your study of the equine foot, your appreciation of structure and function will help you define further questions as you assess the health of your own horse's feet.

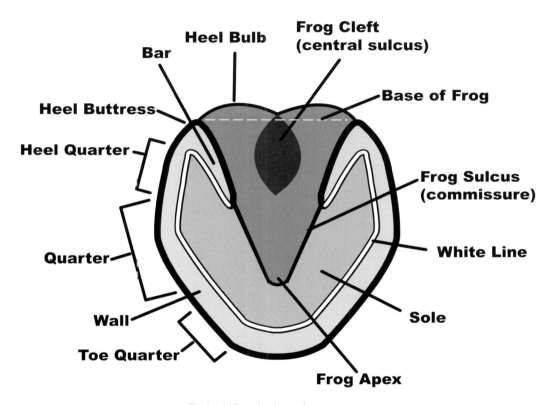

Fig 2.14 Map of solar surface anatomy.

Chapter highlights

- Knowing basic anatomy gives you some information and terminology that will improve communication with your farrier and veterinarian.
- Internal structures of the hoof, such as the coffin bone and the laminae, relate to the outer shape and integrity of the hoof.
- When internal structures are weakened or diseased, often there will be an indication in hoof capsule distortion, such as dished or flared toe wall.
- One of the key surface structures that every horse owner should watch closely is the white line. The white line can give you an early indication of weakening within the hoof. You can inspect it regularly in a bare foot. In a shod foot, remember to look closely during each farrier appointment when the shoes are removed.

Recommended Reading

Color Atlas of the Horse's Foot, Chris Pollitt, BVsc, PhD
Building the Equine Hoof, David M. Hood, DVM, PhD

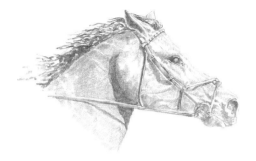

chapter three

Reading the Hoof

- **Evaluating Soundness**
- **Checklist for Hoof Health**
- **Understanding Static Balance**

Horse owners assume a high level of responsibility for the condition of their animals. With this responsibility comes the assumption that you know what your horse needs. To understand the importance of having a sound knowledge base from which to make decisions, think about your relationship with a somewhat less complex item, your car or truck.

You drive every day and the vehicle seems fine. Then one day you notice the steering wheel is beginning to pull just a bit to the right. Your response is determined by how much you know about cars in general and your vehicle's history in particular. If you know a little, you may head to a repair shop, trusting that the mechanic will accurately (and honestly) diagnose the problem. Or you may choose to do nothing until the problem becomes critical.

If you know a bit more, you may decide to look at the tires for additional clues. Are they wearing evenly? Do they have the proper pressure? After a long high-speed drive does one wheel get hotter than the other? All of these are clues that will point to or eliminate the potential sources of the problem. Above all, you know that any change from the normal is worth further investigation.

You may elect for a more proactive approach. You make sure the vehicle has its scheduled maintenance, consistently check tire pressures and tread wear, and regularly track fuel mileage so you can immediately discern changes in your car's health. You also learn the early-warning signs of potential problems so you are never stranded on the side of the road.

When you take a similar proactive approach toward your horse's hoof care and health as you might to a vehicle, you provide the level of knowledge and vigilance needed to make sound decisions regarding your horse.

Evaluating Soundness

What is soundness and how is it evaluated? The simplest answer is that soundness is the absence of limping. Veterinarians evaluate evidence of pain by watching a horse move, conducting joint mobilization and flexion tests, palpating the leg and hoof or using hoof testers. This clinical assessment has obvious value. But there are limits to these conventional evaluation techniques.

In some cases a horse does not appear lame in an exam, but is consistently lame after a few miles of riding. If a horse passes a veterinary soundness test one day, and is lame the next, does this mean he was or was not sound when the vet saw him? There is no answer to this question, yet asking it can broaden our view of soundness. By the time we see a symptom, the cause is likely to have been silently at work for a long time.

A horse that looks sound today is not necessarily free of pathology. Health is more than the absence of textbook medical conditions. Health is not as well understood as disease due to our way of defining disease as the presence of a specific dysfunction that has been scientifically identified. Health is the condition of natural biological function. Health allows an animal to effectively cope with all stress including cuts, scrapes, bruises, broken bones, and infectious illness.

> **Soundness… is an aspect of health, and is more than the absence of limping.**

A sound horse will be able to meet the demands of physical and mental stress. Soundness then, is an aspect of health, and is more than the absence of limping. Since we cannot objectively measure something that we can't see, it is difficult to determine if our apparently sound horse is actually healthy. This leads us to wonder: can we find out if there is underlying damage being done? The next thought may be: can we make our sound horse "more sound?"

The indicators of hoof health discussed in this chapter provide tools to help evaluate horse hoof health. Health can deteriorate when biological structure and function are out of alignment. Structure, how the body parts are held together, is linked to function. Function refers to what the specific parts do to maintain the animal.

If the hoof's ideal structure becomes altered in any way, its function will also be altered. The cause of hoof change can be nutritional, environmental, or mechanical. Any changes to the balance and alignment of hoof components will affect the physiological function. In turn, changes in hoof structure and function will effect changes in structure and function of other parts of the horse's body.

How well any particular horse copes with a life full of challenges and stress is dependent on numerous environmental and genetic factors. Difficulty in identifying, preventing, and curing common equine soundness issues is compounded by controversy regarding how a healthy foot is supposed to look. We need to know the components, the contexts, and the parameters of horse health in order to promote and maintain hoof health. We must search constantly, learning about our own horses and the wider world of equine research in order to understand what will encourage health in these animals. As in all research, there are competing theories, contradictory explanations for a single phenomenon, varying opinions on what constitutes normal, and a multitude of ideas about what we should be doing to reach the goal of soundness.

When considering the advice of experts, do not lose sight of your own knowledge of your horse. Your powers of observation and intuition are valuable. If you ask a farrier why a shoe or foot looks a certain way, and the answer is "that's how it's always done," or "this is what they teach in school" or, "you take care of the riding, I'll take care of the feet…" or any number of other evasive responses, it is up to you to seek answers from other sources. Horse owners are rarely given enough credit for their own hunches. We have all been taught to defer to experts. If you look more closely at the source, you find that much of "expert opinion" is based on custom and habit rather than careful study of horse health.

By gaining an understanding of the concepts laid out in this and the following chapters, you are preparing yourself to be the expert manager of your own horse's health.

Checklist for Hoof Health Evaluation

What does a healthy hoof look like? Most horsemen have a sense of a few indicators of hoof health. For example, if a hoof lacks obvious cracks, flares or bruises and the horse does not limp, we tend to assume the foot is healthy. But what are the possible warning signs of impending hoof problems? Is there a way for horse owners to systematically evaluate multiple aspects of hoof health and anticipate or avoid hoof trouble in the early stages? A complete veterinary exam is one way to get an in-depth assessment of the horse's foot. There are also some simple, non-technological methods that may be used to judge the health of the hoof. While x-rays provide an internal view of the hoof, external anatomy will provide an estimate of hoof health.

Hoof care professionals draw on their education, experience and intuition when assessing a hoof. They draw on multiple clues that reveal the integrity of hoof function such as shoe or hoof wear patterns; quality of horn; shape, symmetry and balance of all four feet. This chapter offers insight into how an experienced farrier assesses your horse. Although farriers may not always agree on what constitutes balance and health in your horse's hooves, this checklist provides a list of topics used by many farriers.

Your thorough study of the hoof will ultimately lead to the development of your own approach to assessment. Hoof evaluation is not limited to the few points discussed here and need not be conducted in the order presented. Experienced farriers assess many of these parameters simultaneously. However, when learning something new, it helps to have a step-by-step approach.

The evaluation begins with the foot as seen from a distance. The checklist then moves to finer details that require picking up the foot and examining it carefully. Farriers tend to look at a horse's feet first, whether they are looking at a client's horse or just observing horses out in pasture. As you become aware of the importance of hoof health, you are likely to find yourself looking at horses from the hoof up.

The culmination of your hoof health assessment is evaluating balance. Hoof health stems from, and results in, balance. This chapter introduces balance, and the concept of balance reappears throughout the book. Be patient as you learn the key components. You will become increasingly more comfortable with the concepts over time.

To identify hoof problems, consider multiple symptoms and think about the big picture of health. Any single indicator can be insignificant or even misleading. You must guard against over-interpreting any single indicator. Practice your skills anywhere you see horses.

The eleven specific areas of assessment in the following checklist will uncover clues about stresses on the hoof. Farriers and veterinarians spend years learning about complex and controversial issues of hoof health and balance. Here, you are introduced to the basic concepts they have studied. This will allow you to take an active and informed role in partnership with your equine practitioners.

1. Movement and Stance

The first item on the checklist for assessing hoof problems is how a horse moves and stands. Horses that trip, land toe first, take short strides, interfere, forge, or display any number of other gait abnormalities may be moving this way because of pain in their feet or elsewhere in the body. There are numerous reasons for poor movement, back or neck pain being common ones. Certain illnesses can cause gait abnormalities so it is important for a stumbling horse to receive a thorough veterinary exam. Hoof health always needs to be checked when your horse exhibits poor movement.

A horse that moves well is not necessarily free of pain. Some horses move well despite a certain level of discomfort. In this case you may have to look for more subtle clues that something is amiss. A sport horse that loves his job may perform very well, but when placed back in his stall or pasture, may display signs of discomfort by standing off balance to compensate for pain.

Examine the way the horse stands. Difficulty standing square, pointing one front foot forward, constantly shifting weight from one front foot to another, or standing splayed out, may all be signs of foot pain. Sometimes a horse moves well for many years but stands in a suspicious manner, such as "parked out" with front legs ahead or hind legs underneath the body. Some horses with foot pain stand with their front legs further underneath, rather than in front of a limb axis perpendicular to the ground. Either deviation can indicate foot discomfort. If the cause of pain is not removed, eventually it is likely to manifest as lameness. Owners who can identify these signs at the stance phase can often correct them before the problem ever clinically affects the horse's movement.

When you pick up a foot, check to see where the horse wants to hold the leg. Lift it gently and wait a moment, feel for the horse's own tension to pull the foot where it most naturally wants to hang. You can gather important information from this simple exercise. If the front foot wants to swing under the horse's belly, this may indicate muscular problems in the triceps and other muscles around the elbow. If the horse wants to cross one hind leg past the other, or can't pull the hind leg out at all and instead drags it under his belly, there may be problems in the hip, hock, or stifle.

If you never pick up the feet you might miss valuable, early cues. Many horses have movement problems or stance irregularities dismissed by owners and veterinarians as meaningless. People convince themselves "that's just the way he is." Yet once the feet are balanced, these abnormalities may disappear.

2. Hoof-Pastern Axis

Start by assessing the axis of the hoof in relation to the pastern. Look to see if an imaginary line drawn through the foot and pastern, parallel to the front of the hoof wall, is roughly continuous. The only way to be absolutely sure if the bones are aligned properly is to see an x-ray. The external view or "eye-ball" method can give you a general idea of bone alignment in the lower limb. Bone alignment is important for biomechanical efficiency, which means a horse will move with as little effort and as little damage to himself as is physically possible.

3. Toe and Heel Length

Hoof length refers to how much wall is present. Farriers commonly remove excess length from around the entire perimeter of the foot or as needed from just the toe or heel. Every horse has an optimum heel-toe length ratio although there are no objective studies to provide guidance. It is important to develop a general

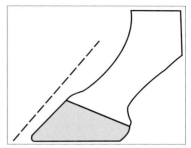

Fig 3.1a Normal hoof-pastern axis.

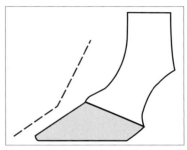

Fig 3.1b Broken-back axis places excess stress in the navicular region.

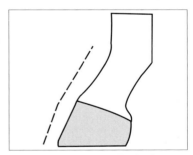

Fig 3.1c Broken-forward axis places excess stress along the dorsal hoof wall.

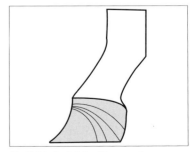

Fig 3.1d A club foot is an extreme version of broken-forward.

appreciation for signs of distortion rather than aim for specific number of inches of hoof wall length.

A long toe is usually easy to identify, particularly if the toe horn becomes dished. A dish is the term used to describe a depression of the toe wall. A slight dish may be a subtle depression in the middle of the hoof wall at the toe or it may include a grossly distorted toe wall that curves up like the tip of a ski.

Long heel is not always easy to see at first glance if it is under-run. Interestingly, a long heel may be commonly interpreted as "no heel" because it is crushed underneath the foot, out of view. In the case of an under-run heel, we observe the heel bulb dropped almost or entirely on the ground. The way to identify long, under-run heel is to look very closely at the wall horn in the heel and quarters. Follow the horn tubules from hairline to the ground: if under-run, the tubule angle will be almost parallel to the ground. If normal, the tubule angle will be more upright, that is, almost, but not quite, parallel to the dorsal hoof wall tubule alignment.

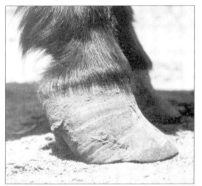

Fig 3.2 Foundered pony hoof after long-term neglect has assumed a club foot conformation with both long toe and long heel.

Long but not under-run heel is easy to see. The horse will look "lifted up" in the back of the foot, like he is wearing high-heeled shoes. Look at the heels from behind the horse, standing on a flat surface. You will see space between the base of the frog and the ground. Sometimes you could stick several fingers in that space. If the whole foot is too long, heel and toe, you'll get the impression that the whole horse is too high off the ground as if he is wearing platform shoes.

Sometimes feet grow long but remain reasonably free from distortion; in such feet a well-trained eye is needed to detect potential problems. Typically, excess length will display noticeable signs such as flares, cracks, or dishing. A flare is usually seen on the sides of the hoof when wall on one side is longer and appears to curve in or out. One crack or even multiple cracks may appear anywhere in the hoof wall but most commonly they are seen in the quarters.

Flaring, cracking, or dishing all suggest that the hoof is out of balance. However, a single piece of evidence is not enough to define the problem. These signs can be present on a hoof that is either too long or too short. How do you differentiate between too long and too short? You look at multiple indicators of balance. After you have read through the rest of this checklist the heel-to-toe ratio will make more sense. For now, keep in mind that an average fifteen-hand horse with a healthy foot will rarely have a hoof length exceeding 3½ inches at the toe.

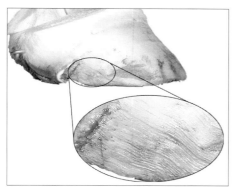

Fig 3.3 This freeze-dried specimen from a foot with a broken back axis shows typical crushing of the heel horn. Close-up view shows horn tubules almost parallel to the ground with the wavy "unraveling" appearance of weak horn.

4. Hoof Shape

The shape of the foot is influenced by both the environment and locomotion behavior. Notice the difference between front and hind foot shapes. Typically, front hooves appear round across the toe while hind feet appear somewhat more pointed.

It is common to see hind feet that look like front feet. One also sees front feet that are narrow and pointy, which look like hind feet. Another deviation is feet that are squared off at the toe. Any of these hoof shapes may indicate a problem with hoof balance and function. However, a deviation from the typical shape does not necessarily mean there is a problem. For example, some barefoot horses will, on hard ground, have slightly squared toes on the front feet, although this may happen only when the feet get too long. The "breakover point" refers to the last part of the foot to leave the ground as the leg moves from weight bearing to the swing phase of the stride. If the natural point of breakover is not exactly centered, most horses do fine as long as the overall imbalance is not exaggerated. Breakover will be discussed in depth in Chapter 4.

When you see hind feet that look like typical round front feet, this may indicate a hind end problem. When horses drag their hind feet, people are often under the impression that this is part of the normal locomotion for some horses. It is not normal for hind feet to be square in the toe or for horses to drag them. If your horse is dragging his feet, consider consulting an equine chiropractor or veterinarian.

Some horses do not naturally move their limbs in a straight plane, even when the feet are well trimmed and balanced. A rider may require the horse to move in a straight line if this will provide an advantage in the show ring. A farrier can deliberately manipulate the trimming, balancing, and shoe placement to cause the horse to move as the owner desires. If the natural hoof shape and therefore motion of the horse is altered for show purposes, it may be detrimental in the long-term. Forcing a horse to move in what appears to be a straight fashion, even if he has inherent limb faults, can do damage to hard and soft tissues of the limbs and feet.

There are different styles of shoeing, some favoring squared off toes. Little research is available to guide farriers on ideal toe shape. A horse may appear to move better or stay sound in the short term with squared toes. However, this is not usually the natural contour of the white line and hoof wall; therefore this special shoeing style should only be applied to your horse with good reason. If your farrier cannot explain to you the reasons for this shoeing style, it might be worth leaving the toe of the foot more naturally shaped.

Many horses have mismatched feet. Horsemen may feel this is normal, that it may be hereditary, and that nothing can or ought to be done about it. In some cases, this is likely to be true. In other cases, mismatched feet can be a warning sign, and something can and should be done.

> **If your farrier cannot explain to you the reasons for this shoeing style, it might be worth leaving the toe of the foot more naturally shaped.**

A lot of horses have one smaller foot. The smaller foot may be an abnormal shape, often more narrow with higher heels. Associated with this foot size difference is often a body asymmetry – shoulders or hips misaligned, rib cage differently shaped on each side, neck or spine curved to one side. Asymmetry is often accompanied by a "sidedness," that is, a preference for turning one way. Some horses always prefer a certain lead, or always go over trotting poles with the same front foot leading. Perhaps the smaller foot is caused by navicular or other pain that makes the horse protect the foot by placing less weight on it, and the consequence is that the foot "shrinks" from less use.

Perhaps these asymmetries are present at birth. They may begin with a crooked rider, or ill-fitting tack, or other possible causes. It is worth close attention because in some cases it can be changed.

If the cause can be attributed to pain in the back of the foot, for example, there may be certain shoeing or trimming methods that can ease the pain or even reverse the condition, in which case the foot can be used normally again. If the cause is due to pain in the body, chiropractic or veterinary treatment may be able to eliminate it.

There are training methods that can help develop body-awareness. Simple changes of habit, such as leading a horse from the off-side, may serve to rebalance the body. The horse will tend to lean toward the handler, and if you always handle your horse from the near side, he is likely to lean a bit towards you and place more weight on the left front foot. Try mounting from the other side, lunging for longer on the other side, or spending more time grooming on the other side.

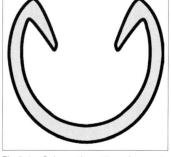

Fig 3.4a Schematic outline of normal front foot.

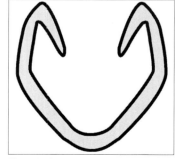

Fig 3.4b Schematic outline of normal hind foot.

5. Hairline

The coronet, also called coronary band, is the junction between hoof wall and hairline at the pastern. In most cases, the hairline will give you some idea of hoof balance. Like all of the indicators discussed in this book, it should not be taken as a single, reliable measure of hoof balance or health. In certain feet the hairlines appear distorted but there is not necessarily internal misalignment. It is worth re-emphasizing, not to place too much significance on one indicator, as there are certain popular methods that interpret hoof balance based only, or primarily, on the hairline.

The hairline on a healthy foot tends to slope toward the ground in a straight line from toe to heel when viewed from the side. When seen from the front, the hairline should be the same distance from the ground on each side. One common distortion is a hairline that is higher on one side, indicating that the coffin bone may be correspondingly tipped to one side. For a good view of this stand in front of your horse and crouch down so you get a "hoof's-eye" view. The horse must be standing on a flat, hard surface such as concrete or a rubber stall mat. Any uneven footing at all, even a dirt area that seems flat, can cause a misreading of this indicator.

Another frequently seen distortion is a hairline that is wavy or bulging upward, usually in the quarters. Farriers often refer to this as a "jammed" coronary band. There is little research on this, and, in fact, some controversy as to whether such a hairline indicates anything significant at all. Many farriers believe that the bulging is caused by an uneven wall length. Often the hairlines "settle," that is, return to a normal straight alignment, after the farrier re-balances the foot. There are times when an imbalance has been present for a long time and although proper trimming may balance the foot, the hairline might not change.

Swelling around the pastern and fetlock can be an indication that the foot and lower leg have been overloaded. Local trauma to these tissues can come from unbalanced shoeing or trimming, in which case you will see the swelling disappear when the feet are in better balance. Swelling can occur when feet are well-balanced; this is usually an indication that the horse is being used beyond his capacity. Getting a horse fit entails some measure of "normal overload." When followed by appropriate rest time, the swelling abates and these tissues can meet higher demands without breaking down.

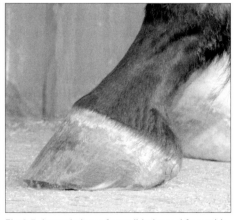

Fig 3.5 Lateral view of a well-balanced foot with straight hairline, straight dorsal hoof wall, good hoof-pastern axis.

A coronet that is chronically swollen and puffy can be a sign of long-term imbalance. The cause can be attributed to improper trimming, or the horse may have a structural imbalance, possibly due to pain, resulting in overload to one side of the foot. If your horse has wind puffs on the medial side at the coronet, check the mediolateral balance. Commonly horses with medial hairline swelling have a low medial wall. Restoring proper balance will result in reduction or even complete disappearance of swelling.

Research on the fluid pressure in the coronary band shows that pressure changes significantly when the horse is in motion and the pressure does not change under weight-bearing when the horse is standing still. However, if the laminae are weakened or the foot has other problems with internal shock-absorbing tissues, one might speculate that the coronary area would receive more force than it was designed to bear, even under static load.

When your farrier has trimmed and shod the horse in balance, and the horse is not worked hard, yet still has puffy swelling in the coronary area, this could indicate internal trauma, perhaps from a previous injury that never healed properly. Whatever the cause, coronary band swelling is not normal, and you should investigate possible ways to alleviate it.

Other coronet problems, such as a hard swelling at the front, or an indentation ledge all the way around the hoof capsule, can indicate founder. The hard swelling can be from the extensor process pushing forward into the coronary groove when the coffin bone rotates. Run your finger around the hairline right at the ridge where the hard hoof capsule meets the soft tissue above it. If you feel a dip or indentation, this can indicate a dropped, foundered coffin bone, commonly called a "sinker."

Swelling in the quarters and around the back of the foot just above the coronary band might be due to damage in the lateral cartilage. Cartilage matrix is connective tissue with water content that results in a gel-like material. It can be of varying stiffness and functions to manage shock in many places in the body. When the cartilage is squeezed, water is pushed out of the cartilage matrix, and water returns as the material resumes its original shape. Hoof cartilage is able to stay resilient and resist compression in order to act as a framework for maintaining the shape at the back of the foot since there are no bony structures beyond the back of the palmar processes.

If the cartilage on either side of the hoof is subject to excess force, it may develop bony deposits, called ossification, and in some cases may ossify completely. When it turns into bone, it is called sidebone. Conventional veterinary medicine considers this inconsequential because many horses have sidebone and it does not usually cause lameness. There is speculation that this tissue is meant to be part of the force-reducing mechanism of the hoof, and sidebone could be a sign of unbalanced, malfunctioning feet.

6. Hoof Wall

Look closely at the texture and color of hoof wall surface. In a healthy hoof the hoof horn is smooth and may even be shiny. Run your fingers over the surface to check for subtle dishes or flares that may not be apparent at first glance. Hoof integrity can be compromised by loads that are too heavy, imbalanced, or both. For example, if a horse injures one leg, the other legs must support more than their share of the load. This will predispose the supporting hooves to flaring or dishing.

When the hoof wall is weak, despite good balance, the wall may crack, chip or flare equally around the bottom edge. If the wall is also off-balance, more distortion will be apparent, such as asymmetrical dishing or flaring. Sometimes a horse with very thin hoof walls will walk entirely on the sole and frog until the whole hoof is healthy enough to grow thicker wall.

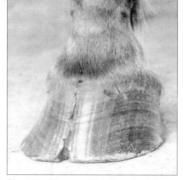
Fig 3.6a Damaged hoof wall with multiple signs of imbalance: wavey growth rings, flaring, dishing, cracking, and distorted hair line.

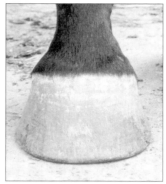
Fig 3.6b Balanced, healthy hoof wall: solid, smooth, no distortions.

The layer of periople just below the coronet can be slightly roughened and turns white. A white color to the periople is normal, and is most visible during wet weather or if the horse is turned out in wet pasture. Sometimes the periople gets inflamed and overgrown. Excess roughness, pitting, or overgrowth of the periople can all indicate health problems within the hoof.

The hoof horn should be smooth with no distortions. A common warning sign of internal dysfunction is wavy growth rings. Like growth rings found on trees, these ridges offer important clues. Often called "fever rings," these ridges indicate times of injury or systemic stress. Outer hoof wall is generated at the coronet and grows downward, usually at a rate of one quarter to one half inch per month in healthy horses. You can estimate when stress occurred by measuring the distance from the coronet to the growth ring.

The rings can provide other information. Follow two neighboring rings from the midline at the toe around until they disappear at the heel. If the space between the two rings gets further apart at the heel, this indicates that the heel has grown faster than the toe. This type of wall distortion is common on feet that are chronically off balance, often due to improper trimming and shoeing. The other common cause of this distortion is

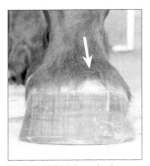

Fig 3.7 Whitish periople visible just below hairline.

chronic founder. All of these signs generally indicate that the foot is experiencing forces it is not designed to bear.

When evaluating the hoof wall, look for signs of hydration problems, which can sometimes mimic balance problems. The horse's hoof does not appear designed to require external sources of moisture. Healthy feet resist moisture changes. Horses can live in swamps or deserts without feet becoming aversely affected. Feet that are unhealthy lack the normal barrier functions of hoof wall, and may be predisposed to drying out or becoming soggy. Feet that crack may be too dry. Feet that flare, don't hold nails well, or have crushed horn tubules may be too wet. Soaking dry feet or "dry-lotting" a horse with wet feet can be a temporary solution in treating symptoms. Look for any underlying cause, because healthy hooves do not need special hoof dressings or soaking on a regular basis.

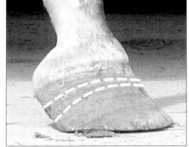

Fig 3.8 Growth rings spaced further apart at heel than at toe, typical of unbalanced foundered feet and most pronounced in feet left too long between trim appointments.

Causes of hoof moisture problems may be nutritional, with a mineral imbalance being one common cause of impaired horn growth and/or function. Horn quality can also be compromised by toxicity, such as selenium poisoning from ingesting certain plants. There may be metabolic explanations for slow or defective horn growth and integrity. Cushing's horses, for example, can have collagen disorders that cause an array of problems, skin and hoof tissue weakness being just one possible manifestation.

7. Solar Surface Proportions

A properly balanced foot has more weight-bearing surface behind the frog apex than in front of it. Be sure to look at the bearing surface because this will be changed by the trim. The reference line at the back of the foot is from heel to heel where the horse lands. In feet that are off-balance because of under-run heels, this line will be well forward of the base of the frog. If there is much more foot in front of the reference line at the frog, the farrier will decide where the foot needs to be trimmed to return the proportions to normal. There are times when the toe needs to be removed, other times heel needs to be removed. In more distorted feet optimum balance may not be achievable in one trim if the horse is to be left barefoot. When the horse must work and there is no time for slowly returning the balance over several trimming intervals, shoe placement can immediately change the bearing surface and improve balance.

8. Frogs

A healthy frog usually appears broad and flat, with narrow clefts along the side and a shallow central cleft. The central cleft should look more like a thumbprint, or a wide dip, rather than a deep narrow crack. The tip of your hoof pick should not disappear into the frog clefts when you are cleaning the feet out.

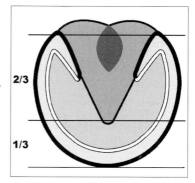

Fig 3.9 Diagram of ideal solar surface proportions. A quick glance at the foot should reveal more bearing surface behind the tip of the frog than in front.

Healthy frogs will vary in consistency depending upon the ground surface. In wet terrain, they will be more "plump" and in dry terrain, they will be leather-like. Unhealthy frogs may be either too big or too small. There are no quantitative studies to tell us exactly what size the frog should be in relation to the rest of the foot. There are qualitative assessments that guide the farrier each time a decision is made to trim back an overgrown frog or rebalance a foot to encourage a change in frog size. Frog atrophy (shrunken) or hypertrophy (over growth) generally happens in conjunction with other dysfunction.

The frog tissue can directly display signs of dysfunction. A frog that is too big will tend to have a swollen appearance, almost as if it is about to burst. The back part of the frog becomes bulbous and is usually soft, sometimes with cracks around the edges. Generally, with such a frog you find under run heels and flared quarters. It is common to see overgrown frogs on flat feet with weak walls. This may be because the frog has overgrown as a way to support the back of the foot when the walls and heels are unable to do so.

Small, sometimes pencil-thin, shrunken frogs are commonly seen. The frog tissue is either rock hard or so squishy that you can stick the tip of the hoof pick deep down into the central cleft. Frogs that are too small are usually found on contracted feet or those with high heels in which the frog has had no ground contact.

In some feet, the frogs become healthier as the back

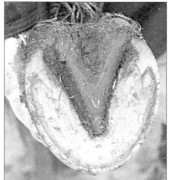

Fig 3.10a Healthy hind foot of a four-year-old Arabian gelding taken in mid-winter. In wet winter weather, the frog has the consistency of a rubber eraser. Notice central sulcus looks more like a thumbprint than a crack. Apex of frog is rounded.

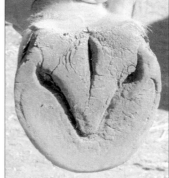

Fig 3.10b Photograph taken in mid-summer of same foot. Notice the frog is wider, flatter, and has a hard, leather-like appearance.

of the foot is lowered closer to the ground. You may not see the frog touching the ground, but this alone does not tell you whether or not the frog is appropriately loaded. Remember that what you see on a concrete floor is not what the foot sees in its normal environment. When the ground is deformable, it will fill in the solar surface and so the frog will effectively be on the ground. But some feet are just too far from the ground, no matter how deformable the surface.

In the neglected foot shown in Fig 3.10c, you can see so much empty space between the frog and ground you could shove several fingers in the space (don't try this!) More important than exactly where the frog sits in relation to the cement floor is the quality of the frog. If it is shrunken, shriveled, and appears non-functional, it is probably not doing its fair share of weight bearing.

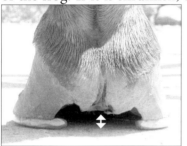

Fig 3.10c A hoof which is overdue for shoeing. Note large space between frog and ground due to overgrown hoof wall.

In general, badly proportioned frogs with poor quality horn tend to appear when the back of the foot is not functioning properly. When the horse's feet receive balanced hoof care, the walls and heels become stronger and more functional, allowing the frog to assume a normal size, shape and consistency.

A central goal of your hoof health assessment is to develop an eye for ideal proportions and horn quality that suggests a foot is able to deal efficiently with the demands placed upon it.

9. Sole

Sole quality is one of the most difficult things for the non-farrier to assess. This takes considerable experience, since there are no simple rules to guide the layperson. However, it is worth introducing you to the concept of sole quality to heighten your awareness of its significance. The sole of the hoof varies tremendously depending on many factors, particularly environmental conditions and terrain. Farriers look for sole that is resilient: neither too dry nor too wet. Sole that is too dry tends to crack and flake. Sole that is too wet is easily depressed by a sharp object such a rock or a hoof pick.

Depth of sole is an indicator that can only be conclusively determined by an x-ray. Indicators of too little or too much sole depth are not easily described. Sometimes when the walls are too long, the sole is also too deep. As discussed above, signs of overgrown wall can be seen. You can assume that if the wall is long the sole might be too thick as well. When a foot has too much sole farriers describe it as retained sole, also called false sole. This means the foot retains or fails to exfoliate excess sole. Feet that are too short will have the opposite problem; there will not be enough depth of sole. This is a difficult problem to correct. Sometimes feet are the correct wall length, but still lack depth of sole which often indicates that the coffin bone is too close to the sole. These horses are usually sore-footed on hard ground.

One sign that may indicate inappropriate depth of sole is bruising in front of the tip of the frog. This can be easily seen on feet that are too short. On feet with retained sole, bruising does not become visible until the farrier begins to remove the outer layer.

Bruising in the hoof wall, which can be seen on white feet, is often noticeable where the hoof wall is flared. When the flares are gone, the bruising grows out along with the wall and does not re-appear at the top of the hoof.

You often hear that thin soles lead to bruising. While this is true, bruising also occurs on soles that are thick with retained horn. Thick soles may offer more protection from rocky ground. But thick soles may be too stiff, and are vulnerable to internal bruising from coffin bone impact. There is no definitive research demonstrating how much or precisely where in the foot movement takes place, but it is generally agreed that some part or parts must move in order to accommodate forces arising from the foot striking the ground. For purposes of the assessment process introduced in this chapter, simply be aware that bruising is not normal. It is a warning sign to which you must respond if you see it on a consistent basis.

Often, sole bruising occurs in horses that never set foot on hard ground and do not come in contact with rocks. For example the term "stone bruise" is used by some people at a racetrack to describe a crescent shaped bruise in front of the tip of the frog. A likely cause of this bruising is the force of impact of the coffin bone against a sole that is not meant to bear this load.

The second type of bruising commonly seen is in the white line and/or the heels. This type of bruise is visible once the shoe is removed. A shoe that is pressing against the sole can cause bruising along the rim of the shoe or in the heels where the white line bends inward to form the bar.

Bruising in the white line at the toe may be from other causes. Many farriers have noticed that long toes appear to result in bloodstains along the stretched white line at the toe caused by tension. Blood staining in the white line at the toe also appears in toes that are very short, such as clubfeet. This is probably because the toe wall has been overloaded by compression. In either case, the bruising may disappear once the foot is balanced.

A shod and padded hoof will move confidently over sharp objects, even to the point where an excessively sharp rock can penetrate a pad. One human response to this is to think that it's good the pad was there or else the damage might have been worse. You could look at it another way. If the pad were not there, the horse might not have put his full weight on something so sharp!

Without added "protection," the horse might not step down with his full weight since a horse's foot can sense the ground beneath. The sensory capability of the hoof means that it provides its own protection. This entails constant signals from the foot sending messages about how much weight can safely be placed on the ground. Think about yourself walking barefoot; if you begin to step on something sharp, you reflexively pull your foot up to avoid applying full pressure.

In short, bruising anywhere on the foot tends to be related to imbalance and should disappear when better balance is achieved.

10. White Line

The white line is the junction between the solar horn and wall horn. Farriers describe a healthy white line as tight and narrow. This is in comparison to an unhealthy white line, which might be stretched and wide. The normal white line on an average sized foot (4½ inches across widest part of the sole) is approximately 1/8th of an inch or less. On a hoof that has been left barefoot, the white line can be seen easily if it is unhealthy. This is because the stretched horn becomes wide and often separates, leaving a depression around part or all of inner hoof wall. A healthy white line on a bare foot forms a seamless connection between wall and sole. For you to inspect it properly, the foot must be free of any dirt. The white line might need to be lightly rasped in order to bring its detail into view.

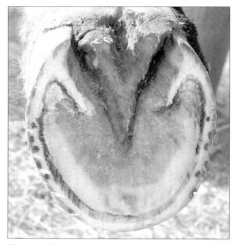

Fig 3.11 Stretched white line showing separation between hoof wall and sole. The rest of the foot looks good: bar, sole, and frog appropriately proportioned.

With a shod horse, make a point to look at the feet during a farrier appointment after the shoes are pulled. In shod feet the white line might appear separated around the nail holes. If the feet are healthy this is a superficial blemish and not a sign of weakness. The separation is rasped or nipped off before the next set of shoes is nailed on.

One warning sign of ill health, possibly laminitis, is a "stretched" or distorted white line that does not improve once the foot has been trimmed. This means the damaged, separated horn is not merely superficial. When the white line is stretching, the hoof is subject to infection and further weakening. Another warning sign is blood staining in the white line, which, when combined with stretching, can indicate more severe imbalance.

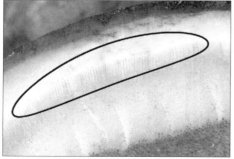

Fig 3.12 Close-up view of good white line with strong connection between wall and sole.

The white line is a useful early indicator of problems as well as health. It is worthwhile for you to pay close attention to this area. If you know the normal width and quality of your horse's white line, you might catch a potential problem before the clinical signs become obvious. For example, if the toe is slightly too long, bruising can develop in the white line. If caught early, the farrier can adjust the balance and by the next appointment signs of bruising may have disappeared. Additionally, if your horse currently has a hoof problem, monitoring the horn quality in the white line can give you some indication of how well the hoof is healing.

The term white line disease has been used to refer to various problems that appear as deterioration of the white line. In some cases there is separation between the white line and the wall, or elongation of the white line, but not necessarily an infection. Research has shown that some cases thought to be infections in the white line are actually a fungus in the hoof wall and this is analogous to nail fungus in humans.

11. Hoof / Shoe Wear

Finally, an experienced farrier looks at hoof or shoe wear to help interpret other signs of hoof health. On shod horses, a farrier will look at both the solar and ground surface of the shoe before re-shoeing a horse. If the steel exhibits asymmetrical wear, balance may be changed in an effort to improve the horse's movement patterns. With barefoot horses, hoof wear patterns provide trim guidance.

Interpreting wear patterns is a complex process. Like tire wear on a car, hoof and shoe wear is used as an indicator of balance, but by itself is not a reliable way to determine where the issues lie. If you see strange wear patterns on your car tires, it may be difficult to tell if the problem is balance, alignment, or flaws in the car's structure. The only thing you can know reliably is that additional assessment is required. The same reasoning applies to hoof and shoe wear.

Understanding Balance

In a dictionary, balance is defined as a "harmonious arrangement of parts." Hoof balance is a concept, an idea. Balance is not easy to capture objectively with a single definition. Harmony of parts describes the essence of hoof balance. If the frog, sole, wall, and bars are correctly proportioned, the foot is likely to be in balance. However, hoof balance is a multidimensional concept, which can be assessed in both static and dynamic form.

Static balance refers to the way the horse loads the foot when standing still. Dynamic balance refers to the horse in motion. Static and dynamic balance are not always the same. A foot may seem balanced when the horse stands still but if the horse interferes, forges, trips or consistently lands harder on one side of its foot, then that horse is not in dynamic balance.

Another definition of balance is "the power or means to decide." In terms of a sport, athletes are in dynamic balance when they are able to move in any direction while staying in equilibrium. A wide receiver in a football game reaches to catch a sideline pass. He wants to stay on his feet and on the field, but since he's not in dynamic balance when he catches the ball, he must go out of bounds to avoid falling. In other words, he is "in balance" going in a direction he didn't want to go. If you are truly in balance, you can move in any direction with ease. To provide a horse with the power to decide exactly where to put his feet is the ultimate challenge of hoof care.

> **To provide a horse with the power to decide exactly where to put his feet is the ultimate challenge of hoof care.**

Understanding dynamic balance and how trimming can affect it is a highly specialized skill. Researchers do not agree on how horses should land. Regarding the mediolateral plane, some believe horses should land level, both heels hitting at once. Other scientists and horsemen believe the horse should land with the lateral heel touching the ground first. There is also no agreement about palmar to dorsal landing. Should the horse land heels first and then roll onto the toe, as humans do? Or should the whole foot come down at once? There is agreement that a pronounced toe-first landing is not good. We do not know exactly how a horse lands on varying terrain, and they land differently at slow and fast gaits.

The human eye cannot resolve the fraction of a second in which the foot is landing. The fine detail of dynamic balance is best assessed using a treadmill and slow-motion video, but it is not certain that what horses do on a treadmill is what they do on other surfaces. Most horse people and farriers do not have access to such technology, thus hoof balance is most commonly assessed in its static form. Currently, static balance is the best indicator of dynamic balance.

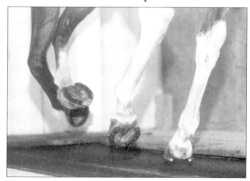

Fig 3.13 Viewing a slow-motion video of hoof landing patterns has shown horsemen that what we think we see in real-time is not always accurate.

Farriers can indirectly gain information about dynamic balance by looking at indicators of how the feet land and bear weight. These indicators include shoe wear, hoof wear, and hoof distortion. If your horse has no distortion in his feet, he is probably landing in a way that appropriately dissipates the forces. The first step to understanding the many aspects of balance is learning to assess static balance. To simplify your study, it is generally safe to assume that the average sound horse in static balance can also achieve dynamic balance.

There are many theories of balance, but most of the work on balance today has been influenced by farrier Dave Duckett, F.W.C.F., widely known for his work on external references of foot and leg bone alignment. Duckett emphasizes the term "horse shoeing," drawing attention to the fact that farriers do not trim and shoe only the hoof, but rather take into account the whole horse, particularly the limb. Duckett's theory is complex, but the basic aim is to trim and shoe for ideal coffin bone and lower leg balance. By finding the center of coffin joint rotation in relation to the outer hoof, the farrier has a guide for hoof horn removal and shoe placement. Getting the foot aligned "from the inside out" puts the foot and limb in the correct position. Optimum hoof and pastern posture then provides the best possible foundation for the whole horse. Efficient stance and movement is the end result of balance according to the Duckett system.

This sounds like common sense. Now, almost two decades after Duckett first presented his findings, the idea of using the bones as a guide for ideal hoof balance has become the standard of care in the farrier industry. There were farriers before Duckett who presented similar ideas and there have been many after him. Yet still many farriers place the shoes on the perimeter of the foot without taking into account the bone alignment. Shoeing merely to "protect" the outer edge of the hoof wall from excess wear remains a widespread practice. Perimeter-only shoeing may appear to work in the short term. But the way to promote ideal hoof balance and to prevent long-term problems is to trim and shoe "the whole horse" with respect to its hoof and pastern alignment.

Familiarity with Duckett's balance theory will give you a benchmark to evaluate other balance theories and provide the needed terminology to discuss balance with your veterinarian and farrier. Duckett's ideas are widely used although no scientific research has actually verified effectiveness. In fact, no scientific research has verified the effectiveness of any particular balance theory. Balance is the part of hoof care that eludes systematic study. You will hear that hoof care is science and art combined. This is true to some extent, but in practice it is largely the art of balance that guides experienced farriers.

> As in many disciplines, science affects the field of hoof care. Readers are urged to learn the basics, but the basics as they are taught to most farriers today have not been the same for centuries. They actually owe a large debt to ideas first presented to the hoof care world in the 1980s, defined by the work of farrier Dave Duckett.
>
> Duckett's work is visionary. Hoof care has been deeply influenced by the insightful changes he created in the way hoof balance is understood and taught. Many have claimed Duckett's work as their own. His ideas are presented so you may appreciate that many practices being promoted by barefoot advocates or in other new hoof theories are built on Duckett's work on breakover and external alignment references.

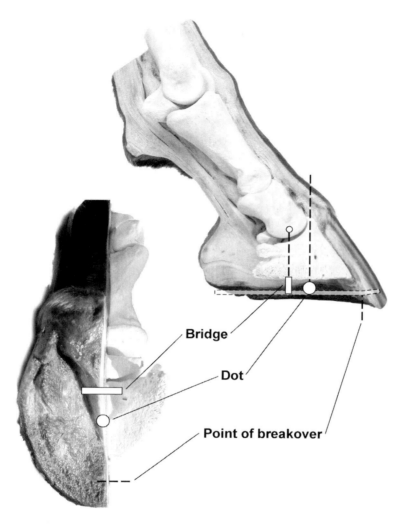

Fig 3.14 Lateral and solar view shows the relationship between internal alignment and Duckett's external references. The Dot marks the center of the coffin bone which lies in the front half of the hoof capsule. The Bridge marks the center of the hoof. A well-balanced hoof will have at least 50% of the weight bearing surface behind the Bridge. The lateral view includes a "mock-shoe" for this specimen to show how shoe placement can be used to balance the foot.

The most well-known aspects of Duckett's balance theory comprise the two external points, the Dot and the Bridge, that help farriers determine ideal foot proportions and optimum shoe placement. The Dot, located about 3/8ths of an inch behind the tip of the trimmed frog, corresponds to the center of the coffin bone. The Bridge, located across the foot at about the bar-frog junction, marks the center of weight-bearing when assessing toe to heel balance.

Duckett found that the Dot is a reference that allows the farrier to determine ideal toe length. The distance from the Dot to the point of breakover should be the same or slightly less than the distance from the medial wall to the Dot. The Bridge is a reference for the center of the weight-bearing surface in the anterior-posterior plane. This reference point is a guide to determine how far back the weight-bearing surface of the bare foot, or the heel branches of a shoe, should extend. Duckett realized that the base of support, the bearing surface of the foot, should have at least as much surface behind the Bridge as in front of it.

To sum up one of Duckett's key guidelines: the Bridge is a less easily identifiable point than the apex of the frog, so a quick and simple method of checking these proportions is to find Duckett's Dot and then identify the solar surface proportions. This guideline was widely publicized by farrier Gene Ovnicek. If you remember only one thing about hoof proportion, remember this: there should be at least 2/3 of the bearing surface behind Duckett's Dot.

It is widely agreed among farriers that "short shoeing," leaving branches shorter than Duckett's suggested length, is poor shoeing, which can unbalance the foot and lead to an assortment of lameness problems. Duckett was an early proponent of what is common knowledge today regarding "caudal support." Duckett's original explanation of this term was that the caudal part of the foot, the portion from the frog bridge to the heels, is designed for weight bearing and concussion reduction. Therefore, the surface area at the back of the foot must be sufficient to support the horse's weight. By trimming and shoeing to increase the caudal surface area, farriers can help to keep feet balanced and sound.

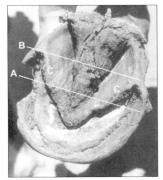
Unbalanced hoof

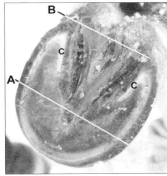
Balanced hoof

Fig 3.15 Compare the solar surface proportions of these two feet. Line A drawn through Duckett's Dot shows that the balanced foot has at least 2/3 of the bearing surface in the caudal part of the foot. The proportions are reversed in the unbalanced foot. Line B identifies the most caudal point of weight bearing. In the balanced foot this line is properly located at the base of the frog. In the unbalanced foot, the heels are so far forward that the landing points are at the level of the navicular bone. The distance between the two lines indicates the effective shock absorbing area of the caudal hoof. The bars are labeled C: note that in the balanced foot the bars end at mid-frog, the location of Duckett's Bridge. In the unbalanced foot, the bars are overgrown and united around the apex of the frog.

Three Dimensional Balance

An important aspect of understanding balance requires appreciation of the foot in three-dimensional space. Duckett's presentations and all of his teachings since the early 1980's have emphasized the essential component of evaluating the foot in multiple dimensions.

Following Duckett's basic concepts, farrier Doug Butler teaches three-dimensional static balance, also called geometric balance. The three dimensions that you can learn to assess are toe-to-heel proportion, side-to-side tilt, and side-to-side mass. For each balance dimension you need to know anatomic terminology and the multidimensional viewpoints of the foot from which you can assess it. Toe-to-heel proportion is dorsal-palmar balance, side-to-side tilt is medio-lateral balance, and side-to-side mass is hoof symmetry.

Dorsal-palmar Balance

Dorsal-palmar balance is an estimation of how well the hoof wall bearing surface is aligned under the limb. This is assessed from two basic views. Lift the foot and observe the solar surface to see how much bearing surface is in front of the tip of the frog compared to how much is behind it. This same proportion can be seen in a side, or lateral, view with the hoof on the ground. From this view you do not know exactly where the tip of the frog is, but you can see if the hoof wall bearing surface looks as if it is under the limb or has grown to extend too far out in front of the limb. (see Fig 3.5 for example of good dorsal-palmar balance.)

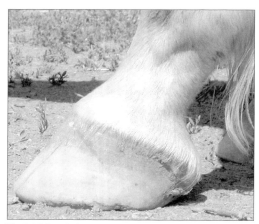

Fig 3.16 Good dorsal-palmar balance.

Medio-lateral Balance

Medio-lateral balance is an estimate of how level the coffin bone is along the solar edge. To assess medio-lateral balance, we need to observe the hoof from two perspectives. First, stand in front of the horse and look at the foot straight on to see if the hairline looks the same height from the ground on medial and lateral sides.

Second, look at the foot from behind the horse. Crouch down to get your eye as close as possible to the level of the heel bulbs. Are the heel bulbs the same distance from the ground? From this view you can check if there is excess heel height.

In a perfectly balanced hoof the medial and lateral solar edges of the coffin bone are parallel to the ground and the hairline is the same distance from the ground on each side of the hoof. There is some natural "play" built into the range of motion of the coffin joint that accommodates movement over uneven terrain. This natural compensation is designed to function as needed from moment to moment but should come back to center when the horse stands on a perfectly flat surface. This compensation helps to preserve soundness, for the short term at least, when the foot is not in perfect medio-lateral balance at the ground surface. For example, during a shoeing interval one side of the wall might grow too long. A certain amount of imbalance of hoof wall horn can exist without compromising the joints further up. But if medio-lateral imbalance is excessive, it can unbalance the joint spaces in the pastern or fetlock. Joint spacing cannot be assessed without x-rays and is mentioned here only to remind you that balance is complex.

Hoof Symmetry

The other aspect of medio-lateral balance is hoof mass, or symmetry. This is observed from three vantage points: solar, anterior or posterior, and top-down. Look for wall deviation. Though few feet are perfectly symmetrical, balanced feet are close to being symmetrical. The most common medio-lateral mass distortion is a flare, which usually occurs on the lateral side of the hoof. Feet can be flared on one side and bent in, or under-run, on the opposite side. Often, asymmetrical feet can be corrected by trimming excess flare. In other cases, inward bent horn is the main distortion and cannot be corrected in a single trimming. These distortions can even out over time and consistent trimming, or, they may need a shoe to be placed where the hoof horn is missing.

Be aware of an important distinction between the two types of medio-lateral imbalance. Some feet with asymmetry are tilted. Generally if a flared foot is neglected for a long time, it will become tilted to some extent. But tilt and asymmetry do not necessarily occur together. A foot may be tilted so that one side is higher, but remain symmetrical in terms of mass on each side. Or, a foot with uneven mass and a very noticeable difference between medial and lateral symmetry may still have a level coffin bone.

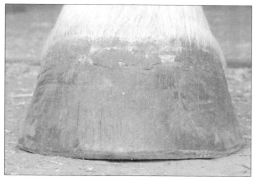

Fig 3.17a This hoof has good medio-lateral balance and is also fairly symmetrical.

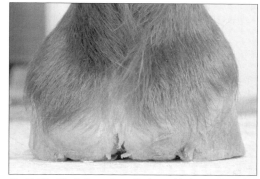

Fig 3.17b Heel view of medio-lateral balance. Stand your horse on a firm surface and crouch down to see a good "coronet eye-view."

In sum, all balance research and opinion since the early 1980's owes some credit to the work of farrier Dave Duckett. There is agreement and disagreement as in any field of applied study. There are researchers and farriers who have focused mainly on the Dot, others on the Bridge, others take into account the whole picture as Duckett continues to teach. As an educated horseman, it is important that you are familiar with Duckett's teachings on the multidimensional relationship between inner bone alignment and outer reference points.

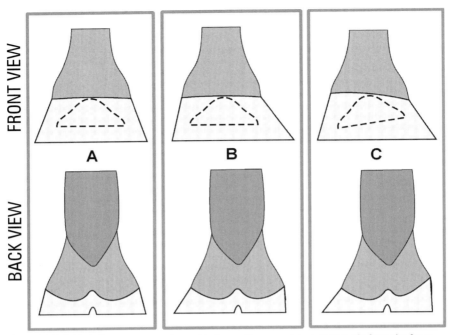

Fig 3.18A,B,C Variations on symmetry and balance. Top row shows schematic from the front, bottom row shows same foot from a heel view. Without x-rays, you cannot be sure about coffin bone position, though there are some general trends that can be estimated from hoof capsule shape.

(A) Medio-lateral balance and symmetry, P3 level.

(B) Asymmetrical foot but P3 still level.

(C) A common distortion in neglected feet. One wall (usually medial) is straight with distorted heel bulbs. Opposite wall flared, and coffin bone tilted. In chronically off-balance feet the hairline is often no longer a useful guide to coffin bone position. In this schematic, the side with the "jammed up" hairline the bone is tilted lower than normal. A foot like this should not be trimmed to make hairlines appear even.

Chapter Highlights

- An 11-point assessment of hoof health begins with close inspection of the following markers of hoof strength, alignment and integrity: hoof-pastern axis; toe and heel length; hoof shape; hairline; hoof wall; solar surface proportions; frog quality, sole quality, white line, and hoof wear pattern.
- To follow discussion and new developments about hoof balance, start with the basics – Duckett's methods.
- Recognizing your horse's basic stance and movement patterns provides important clues to pain in the feet or body.

Recommended Reading

Shoeing in Your Right Mind, Doug Butler, PhD
Maximum Hoof Power, Cherry Hill and Richard Klimesh

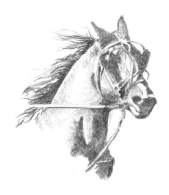

chapter four

Hoof Care Research and Theory

- **The Nature of Research**
- **Hoof Deformation Research**
- **Breakover**
- **Four-Point Trim and Natural Balance**

Your appreciation of hoof balance will be enhanced by familiarity with research on hoof deformation, breakover, natural balance, and four-point trimming. Each of these concepts is complex and they often mean different things to different farriers. If you understand the basics, and are able to "talk shop" with hoof care professionals, you will be well equipped to make hoof care decisions for your own horse.

The Nature of Research

Understanding the benefits and risks of shoeing requires some knowledge of the published research on hoof physiology in relation to shoeing. When assessing research claims, be wary of unwarranted conclusions. The term scientific can be used loosely. The expression "farrier science" implies that farrier methods have been the subject of scientific research. However, most farriers will tell you that shoeing horses is more art than science. Custom, habit, and convention are the mainstream guidelines for how to trim and shoe horses. *Adam's Lameness in Horses*, a standard reference book on equine lameness states: "horses are usually shod on the basis of tradition and not on the basis of scientific study."

When you hear claims such as "a recent study shows that a certain type of shoeing is best for laminitis," find out more about the study before asking your farrier to apply that particular technique. When research horses are shod with a certain type of shoe and they all walk off sound a few of the questions needing to be asked are:

- How were those same horses weeks, months, or years later?
- If the study was conducted over time, was frequency of farrier appointments one of the tested variables?
- Was there a control group of horses that underwent a different type of shoeing?
- Was there a control group that was barefoot?
- How much of the increased soundness could have been due to the trimming rather than the shoeing?

- How much improvement might have been related to the trimming in addition to the shoeing?
- Are other factors or variables considered such as: environment, feed, changed workload, age, use and breed of horses studied?

To answer to these questions a study would need to be well designed with many horses divided into different treatment categories and evaluated over a long period of time. It is unlikely that anyone could receive the funding and other resources needed for a study of this magnitude on trimming or shoeing. Even though these questions probably cannot be answered easily, asking them can help to clarify shoeing concerns and options.

Ask yourself how you know certain things about the horse's hoof. Ask your equine practitioners how they know what treatments are best. What you will find is that much of the customary wisdom is so ingrained that people have never asked where it comes from. Research highlights are included throughout this book because you are urged to "question authority" – explore the sources of what is thought to be gospel.

Hoof Deformation Research

A thousand pounds of horse hits the ground hard when running. How does the horse absorb this kind of natural shock? Normal deformation of the hoof plays an important role. The research on hoof physiology and shoeing over the past century has focused on the related concepts of hoof expansion and shock absorption.

It will be helpful to understand the following common terms used in hoof research: deformation, strain, stress, and elasticity.

Deformation means that if you push or pull on something, it changes shape. Elastic deformation means that the material returns to its original shape when the force is taken away. Plastic deformation means that the hoof did not return to its original shape when the force was removed. When we say, "that hoof looks deformed" we mean it appears to be disfigured. In mechanics studies, deformation is the objective term used to describe movement of a material, like that of an elastic band that changes shape when force is applied.

Strain and Stress

In mechanics, strain is defined as change in length divided by original length. Strain measures deformation. Strain, in this sense, does not mean that there is an uncomfortable amount of movement. Additionally, strain does not mean doing something that is difficult. Neither is strain in the hoof necessarily bad, it is simply an objective measure of how much deformation is present under different conditions.

Hoof research investigates various forms of stress classified as compression, tension, torque and shear. Stress is defined as the force per area. Stress describes the type of force. Strain quantifies the deformation that results from the applied force.

In biomechanics research, the horse's hoof is considered elastic, which means that it springs back to its original shape after being deformed by weight bearing. Elasticity is a theoretical assumption that allows mathematical modeling of the hoof. Perfectly elastic material behaves like a spring, returning the energy rather than losing it as heat. Farriers see hooves changing shape over time and thus describe hoof material as plastic, rather than elastic. Plastic material does not return completely to its original shape when forces are removed.

Well-balanced hooves appear elastic because they maintain a consistent form. Weak or off-balance feet seem plastic because they suffer micro-fractures and do not return to their original shape. A healthy hoof will undergo elastic deformation – expanding under load but then returning to the same unloaded shape when the load is removed.

Farrier texts, as well as hoof research papers, have long stated that the hoof, by design, must be able to reduce the forces of impact. The following mechanisms have all been proposed as contributing to force attenuation: shape changes in the hoof capsule; shape changes in the coronary band; shape changes in the white line; compression of individual spiral horn tubules; pressure changes in the foot's blood supply; and, movement of the cartilage of the foot.

Despite the common assertion that the foot is some sort of hydraulic shock absorber and a pump for the blood, details of the mechanical function are still not well understood. Only in the past few decades have researchers begun to systematically map the intricate workings of force reduction, or shock absorption, in the horse's foot.

Brief History of Hoof Deformation Research

Professor A. Lungwitz recorded the hoof capsule response to bearing weight in the 19th century. Lungwitz found that the hoof capsule moves in the following way when the horse bears weight: the heels expand outward, the front of the coronary band moves back and down and the coronary band around the side and back of the heels expands outward; the bulbs, frog, and sole sink down as the arch of the foot flattens.

Lungwitz noted that each of these movements was small, most were less than half a millimeter. These measurements were assessed on the shod hoof because the shoe was part of the recording apparatus. Subsequent research using different recording devices in both shod and unshod feet has confirmed Lungwitz's findings. Lungwitz commented that an "extensive range of movement" did not occur because "minimal changes of form suffice" for healthy hoof function.

Lungwitz also emphasized that the hoof is never at rest and that the constant shifting and pressure changes are a normal part of the hoof physiology. Describing the coronary band he wrote, "The coronary edge resembles a closed elastic ring, which yields to every pressure, even the most gentle, of the body-weight, in such a way that a bulging out at any one part is manifested by an inward movement at another part."

A century later, in the early 1980s, British researcher and veterinarian Chris Colles demonstrated that the amount of heel expansion did not differ noticeably in shod versus unshod feet. Colles found the expansion distance to be two to three millimeters per heel. In the shod foot, strain was lower and expansion occurred faster. This might indicate that strain was lower in shod feet because other parts of the wall, aside from the heels, did not have as much movement.

While a large amount of hoof wall movement is not necessary to deal efficiently with impact force, the movement of the internal parts of the foot, although difficult to measure, seems to play a significant role. A study published in 1994 by Dyhre-Poulsen compared shod and unshod dampening forces of the digital cushion. Impact vibration measured on the inside of the foot was higher in a shod hoof.

Movement of the coffin bone is even more difficult to measure than movement of the hoof wall. Coffin bone movement correlates with outer hoof wall deformation. Dr. Doug Leach's 1980 dissertation on structure and function of the hoof wall reviewed published reports on hoof wall deformation and coffin bone movement. A handful of studies since then have confirmed the earlier reports, but it remains for future research to reveal the details and variation across the horse population. The normal standing horse has a slight upward slope to the back half of the coffin bone so that the palmar processes are above the level of the distal tip of the bone. There is slight downward movement of the back part of the coffin bone during full weight bearing at the point when only one foot is on the ground during mid-gallop. This range of motion may be an important part of shock absorption. Horses with coffin bones parallel to the ground, or tilted backward slightly, are often unable to work hard without becoming foot-sore.

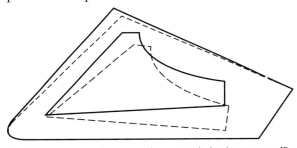

Fig 4.1 Lateral view demonstrating a correlation between coffin bone and hoof wall movement. Solid line shows unloaded hoof, dotted line shows loaded hoof. Illustration depicts exaggerated range of motion.

Research has found that impact vibration is also dampened in the laminar junction, which is the connection between the hoof wall and P3. This finding suggests that inflamed or disintegrated laminar attachments, seen in laminitic horses, would mean that shock would not be effectively dissipated before reaching the bony column. Perhaps joint disorders above the foot can be caused or exacerbated by weak feet that are unable to perform the function of reducing impact forces.

In one experiment, a pressure-recording device was surgically implanted inside the foot, within the digital cushion. The study found a negative pressure, meaning a suction force may exist inside the foot during weight bearing. The negative pressure was

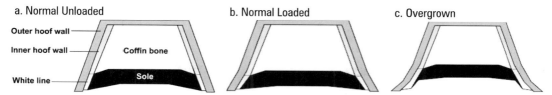

Fig 4.2a, 4.2b, 4.2c Schematics indicating hoof wall movement. (a) Hoof trimmed to level of sole plane has no distortion when unloaded, and (b) minimal distortion in the wall below the coffin bone during loading, returning to normal when unloaded. (c) Overgrown hoof has visible distortion even when unloaded, because the hoof has become "plastic" and exceeded the limits of normal function. The further the wall is allowed to grow beyond the sole plane, the more the wall will be prone to permanent distortion.

found to exist for a longer period of time in the unshod foot. Be aware that at present, conclusions from this study are tentative. The negative pressure testing was done on a few horses and to date no researcher has published a replication of the experiment. We do not yet know if these findings represent the general horse population, or to what extent healthy versus unhealthy feet will show varying pressures in the digital cushion.

Research has shown that an unshod foot has a longer duration of breakover. This suggests that shod feet, because they break over faster, have less time for the hooves to dissipate the energy of impact.

Linking energy dissipation in the foot to breakover, findings suggest that cartilage may ossify in shod feet because the forces on them are abnormal during breakover. When the foot is going from landing to stance to swing phase, it is designed to gradually flex, similar to a human foot going from heel to mid-foot to toe. The cartilage and ligaments that attach to the coffin bone move gradually throughout the limb cycle. In a steel-shod foot breakover happens faster, stretching the cartilage and ligaments forcefully at impact so that they "snap" back as the foot leaves the ground rather than moving back into place more slowly when the stance phase is prolonged, as it would be in the unshod foot.

Only a handful of studies have documented comparisons between expansion in shod and unshod feet. Currently, there is not enough evidence from which to draw firm conclusions about the extent or importance of visible amounts of expansion in standing or slowly moving horses.

Steel-shod feet receive higher impact forces than unshod feet, but the significance of this fact depends largely on the terrain. Horses working on a dirt or turf surface may have little to no negative effects from the impact of steel shoes. Regarding the claim that shoes restrict expansion: steel shoes do appear to restrict expansion to some extent. Again, it is not known whether or not this is significantly detrimental in well-balanced feet.

Breakover

The research community knows very little about breakover and it is a hotly contested topic in biomechanics. The term breakover is used in two separate but related ways. In biomechanics, breakover is the duration of time from when the heels leave the ground to when the last point of the toe leaves the ground. The other sense in which the term breakover is used refers to an actual location on the foot, the last part of the toe wall or shoe to leave the ground. You hear the expression "move the breakover back." This means that the foot is trimmed or shod so that the last point to leave the ground is moved in a caudal direction on the foot; that is, the breakover point is moved closer to the apex of the frog.

The controversy over breakover is about shoe placement, shape, weight, and material. How do you know if the toe is too short or too long? Should the shoe be set flush with the toe or set back underneath it? As discussed in Chapter 3, there are signs from hoof capsule distortion, to sole bruising, to stretching at the white line that can suggest whether the toe is too short or too long. But in general, it can be difficult to tell because we ask so many different things of our horses. Maybe a jumper needs one thing and a dressage horse another. If a horse needs one shoe placement for running about the pasture with his herd and another for the sport you do, you must decide how to compromise.

Breakover Research

Since the 1980s, ideas about breakover and hoof balance have been influenced by Dave Duckett's investigation of hoof biomechanics which revealed reference points on the outer hoof that correspond to internal structures. Duckett's widely known principles, introduced in the previous chapter, are reviewed here because an educated horse owner must understand this shared hoof care language. Duckett's Dot is an external reference point marking the center of P3. Duckett noted what others subsequently observed: "In the unshod foot in a natural environment similar to the arid plains in which the horse evolved, the natural breakover point is maintained." Domestic horses, unable to maintain their natural breakover, must be assisted with good hoof care practices. In 1988, Duckett noted: "if the toe length exceeds these normal parameters, the stresses imposed by the leverage of the unbalanced foot induce injury when the limits of compensation are reached."

Many consider use of Duckett's principles to be the industry standard for shoe placement today. Noted farrier, author, and hoof care educator Doug Butler, PhD states that Duckett's system "varies very little between feet...and it is a true indicator of the position of the skeleton in relation to the hoof base." Duckett dissected hundreds of cadaver feet of domestic horses and found the reference points to be an objective guide to internal bone alignment.

The other important part of Duckett's theory involves the frog bridge, or later called simply "the Bridge." The Bridge is a reference point that corresponds to the center of rotation of the coffin joint. When there is more toe in front than heel behind this point, trimming and/or corrective shoe placement can be used to optimize the bearing surface. If x-rays are not available, the method of locating the Bridge from external points is usually sufficient: one-half to three-quarters of an inch behind the Dot, which is usually the widest point and also is where the bars end about mid-way down the frog. These reference points are reasonably consistent in normal feet. In laminitic or otherwise unbalanced feet, the widest part of the foot is often further forward, and the bars join the frog further forward than they do in a well-balanced foot.

Independent support for the use of the Bridge as a reference point was documented prior to Duckett's work, in 1983, by Dr. Chris Colles. Colles used the radiographically determined reference point from the center of coffin joint rotation to bisect the bearing surface.

There have been no formal scientific studies to confirm or refute Duckett's findings. It is not yet known to what extent these external points correspond to internal points on different shaped feet. Some proponents of natural hoof care believe that the reference points are not constant in naturally trimmed bare feet, domestic shod feet, wild horse feet, laminitic feet, and so on.

To date, only one published commentary casts some doubt on the universal validity of Duckett's theory. Farrier and barefoot advocate Jaime Jackson challenged Duckett's findings in an article published in the *American Farriers Journal*. Jackson took measurements of a wild horse cadaver foot and compared the balance of that foot to Duckett's measurements. Jackson found that the center of balance in this naturally adapted specimen was different. Jackson located the Dot, and then followed a line up through the soft tissue and found it did not exit through the extensor process, but rather was anterior to the exit point predicted by Duckett's theory. Jackson concluded that Duckett's findings are derived from mal-adapted feet and that in healthy feet, the Dot corresponding with the center of P3 would be further back.

A single wild horse specimen was used by Jackson to challenge Duckett's theory. While this cannot constitute evidence for dismissing the significant foundation of clinical confirmation of Duckett's theory of domestic horse feet, it does suggest that more research comparing shod versus unshod, and healthy versus unhealthy feet is necessary before we can claim that we understand what balance should be on all horses.

Studies on breakover from both wild and domestic horses help to clarify external and internal reference points for improving hoof balance. Research on American wild horses has shown that the point of breakover is further back than it is on many domestic horses. Farrier Gene Ovnicek's work on wild horses revealed that the point of breakover was approximately one to 1½ inches in front of the tip of the frog.

Veterinarian Barbara Page's work complements and expands Ovnicek's wild horse research. Page studied clinical application of breakover mechanics and found that using radiographs to determine ideal breakover is an objective and reliable method. Page's work identified several benefits of achieving proper breakover. Comparing feet before and after trimming or shoeing for correct breakover, Page found the following advantages to improve soundness: hoof pastern axis alignment between P2 and P3 improved; the navicular bone moved to a more proximal position in the hoof capsule, thus being under less weight bearing force; there was a decrease of the strain force to the deep digital flexor tendon at its insertion point.

Four-Point Trim and Natural Balance

Reference to the four-point trim means different things to different farriers, which becomes confusing for the horse owner seeking clear definitions. Farriers agree that a short toe with breakover close to the frog apex is part of a four-point trim. Beyond this, characteristics vary depending on the farrier's preference. Additional characteristics of the four-point method may include some, all, or none of the following: low heels, quarters rasped (floated), square toes, shoes set back with toe wall extending beyond the shoe edge. A distillation of the origins of this popular expression may help make sense of current debates.

Gene Ovnicek, farrier and hoof researcher, used the term four-point trim in the late 1980's. In his studies of wild horses, Ovnicek noticed a distinctive wear pattern. High points existed on the hoof wall at the heels, and on the sole across the toe, just inside the white line. Working independently of Ovnicek, veterinarian and farrier Ric Redden also noticed this four-point pattern on barefoot thoroughbred brood mares.

Those who had studied the wear pattern hypothesized that all horses could benefit from variations of a similar trim, naming it the four-point trim. Both variations of this trim featured breakover guidelines first presented by Duckett, in which the breakover point was closer to the tip of the frog than what was popular at that time.

Ovnicek began to describe his method as Natural Balance shoeing. Natural Balance guidelines rapidly evolved, and Ovnicek's system was no longer the four-point trim. For example, when preparing a foot for shoeing, the Natural Balance guidelines advocate leaving the quarters level, rather than lowering, or "scooping" out the wall as was observed in wild horse feet.

Ovnicek also reminded farriers that the toe wall could be left in a natural rounded shape where excess wall hangs over the edge of the square-shaped shoe. Ovnicek's system is based on trimming to the sole plane at the base of the frog. Additionally, Ovnicek emphasizes that farriers should not remove the "toe callus" and should use the knife sparingly, if at all, in front of the tip of the frog.

The term four-point trim today seems to best describe the system developed by Dr. Ric Redden. In contrast to Natural Balance methods, Redden prefers to place the breakover point closer to the tip of the frog, and strives to achieve more foot mass. He has countered reports of unsuccessful application of the four-point trim by suggesting that some farriers may have trimmed to his guidelines after having already done a "regular" trim. If this is done, according to Redden, too much foot was probably removed.

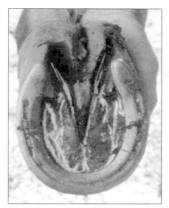

Fig 4.3a Before Natural Balance shoeing.

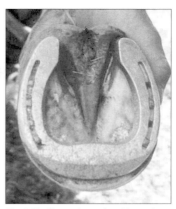

Fig 4.3b Same foot after Natural Balance Shoeing. The shoe is set back behind white line and toe edge is left hanging over the shoe.

In 1997, researcher and veterinarian David Hood tested the four-point hypothesis under controlled conditions. Research determined that the characteristic high points were most likely a product of horses living on soft ground. When horses having the four-point pattern were kept on a hard surface such as concrete, the four points rapidly wore down, leaving the hoof in a much more conventional pattern. Hood's conclusion was that the wear pattern on the hoof wall was due to "ground surface abrasion, and as such is the mirror of true solar loading".

The synthesis of the most convincing research and experience seems to state that the four-point pattern is the result of bare hooves on soft ground. The harder the ground, the less an unshod hoof will exhibit this pattern. Simply stated, the hoof wears most where the load is highest. There is little scientific support for applying a four-point trim under most conditions, especially if the horse is barefoot on hard ground or in shoes.

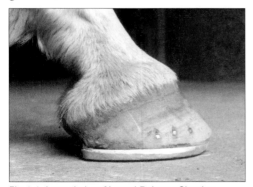

Fig 4.4 Lateral view Natural Balance Shoeing. Shoe placement corrects solar surface balance proportions by moving breakover further back behind the free toe edge.

An offshoot of the four-point trim is the square toe on all four feet. Again driven by observations of wild horses, the square toe has become another method developed to move the breakover point back. Yet not everyone who studied wild horses has observed square toes. Jaime Jackson studied wild horse feet and found they had round front feet and pointy hind feet.

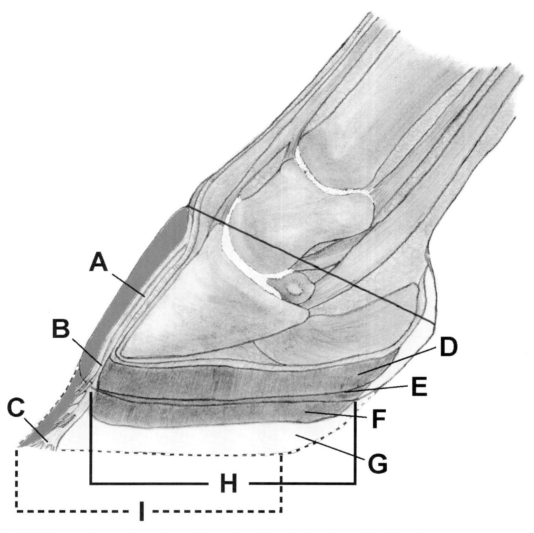

Fig 4.5 Sole plane drawing. Comparison of trimmed (solid lines) and untrimmed (dash-lines) hoof. Artist's rendition of inner hoof with laminar corium and lateral cartilage removed to reveal alignment between hoof capsule and bones.
(A) Laminar junction connecting hoof wall to coffin bone.
(B) Laminar junction below the bone turns into the white line, connecting sole to wall. Connection is tight in the trimmed hoof.
(C) In the untrimmed hoof, white line below the sole plane becomes stretched, distorted, and frayed.
(D) True sole extends almost to the ground in the trimmed foot.
(E) Sole plane – proximal sole is considered "live" and will not exfoliate in a healthy foot. Sole distal to this level may slough off, be removed by the farrier, or become retained.
(F) False (retained) sole accumulates if foot is neglected and grows very long.
(G) Untrimmed wall grows forward away from base of support.
(H) Base of support at level of sole plane. Note caudal-most point of heels is near the back of the digital cushion.
(I) Base of support well below sole plane in overgrown hoof. Wall extends even beyond retained sole. Caudal most points of heel are under the navicular bone

A square toe is contrary to one of the principal tenets of balance by forcing the hoof and horse to move in a certain manner. A square toe forces the breakover to happen parallel to the squared edge of the hoof, which can lead to joint or soft tissue repetitive stress injury.

While squared toes may be helpful for certain hoof or gait issues, the white line determines the natural shape of the hoof. The white line indicates that front feet are round, hind feet are pointy, neither front nor hind feet are square. This does not mean the square toe is always bad. It may be helpful for your horse, but you need to understand the justification for it if your farrier suggests squared toes.

Breakover, four-point trimming, and natural balance all pertain to both trimming and shoeing, so it is valuable for any horse owner to understand and be familiar with these terms.

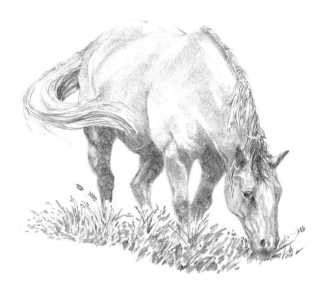

Highlights
- Research is a powerful tool and knowing the validity of the scientific claims is important.
- Following the history of a hoof care trend helps highlight the assumptions that are made without much valid research to support them. Additionally, other groundbreaking methods and theories emerge from a scientific look at many of these assumptions.
- Being a conscientious custodian of your horse requires that you do some research of your own. Whether it is a new miracle shoe, a trimming method guaranteed to prevent lameness or an emphatic statement made by a guru in the industry, don't be afraid to let your instinctive curiosity drive you to find out more.

Recommended Reading
No Foot, No Horse, Gail Williams and Martin Deacon
New Hope for Soundness, Gene Ovnicek

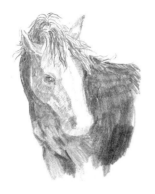

chapter five

To Shoe or Not to Shoe

- **Does Your Horse Need Shoes?**
- **Balance**
- **Hoof Contraction**
- **Pros and Cons of Barefoot**
- **Discussion with Your Farrier**
- **Breaking the Cycle of Pain**

A question asked with increasing frequency in the horse world today is: "Does my horse need shoes?"

When asked what is best, most farriers will answer: "it depends." Experience has shown that some horses perform at their best barefoot. Others perform without shoes but not as well as they would with shoes. There are other horses that need shoes to perform at all. Unfortunately, there is no quick and easy answer for all horses. If you are considering the issue of shoeing versus barefoot, or barefoot rehabilitation if your horse is lame, this chapter offers some facts to consider as you make hoof care decisions.

What distinguishes a horse that can perform barefoot from one that cannot? As with so many questions about feet, the answer depends on a lot of factors including hoof health, terrain, and demands of the particular sport.

Conventional wisdom often urges you to shoe when the feet are weak, flat, have thin walls, tend to chip or flare, or have diseases such as laminitis or navicular. Experience from holistic hoof care professionals has led to the opposite recommendation: barefoot rehabilitation can restore strength and resiliency to the weakest feet. In fact, holistic hoof care professionals tend to recommend that only strong-footed horses be shod. In other words, the ideal candidate for shoeing is a sport horse with no hoof problems, only needing shoes to protect the feet from excess wear or to increase or reduce traction. A weak-footed horse may be better off remaining barefoot and being rehabilitated to full hoof strength before returning to hard work. If the horse cannot afford time off, a weak foot will often be serviceably sound when shod.

A statement about a particular horse needing shoes must be understood in the context of what the rider expects of the horse. During the initial phase of being barefoot, it is common for many horses to experience soreness. If you expect the horse to perform that week or month or even that season, you might reasonably conclude that he needs shoes. If you are able to give the horse time off to adjust to being barefoot, eventually you might find the horse no longer needs shoes. Some horses need only a few weeks of adaptation before they are as sound as they were in shoes. Others may need months or even years before they are comfortable working on hard terrain barefoot. Many horses actually become even more sound barefoot than they had been in shoes. If it takes years to achieve, owners may find it unrealistic or impractical.

There are times when people find that no matter how many different types of shoes and trim preparation techniques are utilized, the horse is lame in shoes. Given this, a barefoot rehabilitation might offer one more chance for recovery.

Many horse owners have found that the choice is not so much shoeing versus barefoot, but rather when and under what conditions different hoof care programs maximize performance and hoof health. Because there is little research on long-term effects of either shoeing or barefoot hoof care programs, the owner must use a logical trial-and-error approach for each horse.

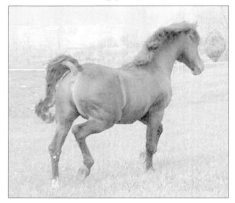

Can shoeing be harmful? The answer depends upon a number of variables: quality of hoof; skill of the farrier; and, how the horse is expected to perform. There are no definitive scientific studies to suggest that shoes harm correctly shod feet. But feet do sustain damage from poor shoeing, or even from good shoeing that is not done frequently enough to maintain balance. Some feet can recover from trauma or disease faster when unshod. Horses living and working on soft terrain, whether they are shod or unshod, may never show any lameness problems. They may have slightly, or even extremely distorted feet, suggesting compromised hoof function, but may never show visible signs of distress as long as they remain on soft pasture and soft riding arenas. Each horse must be assessed individually.

A horse may be able to do some work barefoot; but the mark of top athletes is consistency of performance for years on end. Completing a single event barefoot, such as an endurance race over rough ground is certainly an accomplishment, but can that horse repeat this performance many times per season without going lame? And, would that horse consistently be a top ten finisher? It is one thing for a long-distance horse to go 100 miles in 20 hours; it is quite another to do it in nine hours, as the winners routinely do. It may be that hoof horn simply cannot be replaced as quickly as it is worn off in a demanding high-speed, hard ground, long-distance race. It is yet to be determined if top athletes in challenging hard-terrain sports can remain simultaneously barefoot and consistently sound over an entire career, though it may be possible.

Presently there are many horse trainers who are leaving their horses barefoot and seeing how they perform in different disciplines. Starting a horse barefoot may allow him to continue that way. When a horse has reached competition level in shoes and the owner is not able to give him time off to adapt to a new hoof care regime, keeping him shod may be the most reliable method for ensuring comfort, capability, and consistent soundness.

In deciding to have your horse shod you maintain an obligation to understand the type of trim, the kind of shoes, and the theories and practices to which your farrier is committed. Do not accept a particular type of shoe simply because that is the style of shoeing a farrier does. Find a farrier who will take the time to explain why a certain shoe type is suggested for your horse so that you can make an informed decision.

Balance

As discussed in Chapter 3, balance is crucial to hoof health. Hoof balance is so important that to focus on shoeing versus barefoot misses the big picture. Recall from previous chapters that hoof balance is defined as harmony of parts. Each component of the foot – frog, sole, hoof wall, bar – exists in proportion for maximum efficiency. When any one component is too long, too short, tilted sideways or in any other way distorted, the foot is not in balance and cannot perform ideally.

You may hear of a new shoe on the market and many horses are reported to become more sound with its application. Ask the question: is the improvement from the shoe, or is it from the trim guidelines that go along with that shoe? You can ask the same question of trim techniques touted as unique for barefoot horses. Many of the barefoot trim techniques reported to return horses to soundness are simply good trim guidelines that would return a horse to soundness even if shoes were applied after the trim. The point is, what helps a horse is the technique and timing of the trimming, whether special shoes are applied or not.

> **…what helps a horse is the technique and timing of the trimming, whether special shoes are applied or not.**

Trimming is the foundation of balance. In some cases, balance may be difficult to achieve by trimming alone. For example, when a horse's foot is badly distorted, it can be difficult to correct the imbalance right away. When a horse needs to perform, a shoe may be indicated to give the horse an appropriate weight-bearing surface.

Horses can be unsound and off-balance, whether shod or barefoot. This indicates the need to complete a comprehensive assessment of balance. Until you have conducted a thorough balance evaluation, you cannot draw valid conclusions about whether your horse should be barefoot or shod.

If your horse has balanced feet in shoes, you might find he has no difficulty being barefoot. It is probably worthwhile to see if your horse is as comfortable barefoot as he is shod. It could lead to even healthier feet and save you the cost of shoeing.

If your horse is lame in shoes, even when well balanced, removing the shoes may or may not result in long-term soundness since there are other factors involved. Consider a barefoot approach. It is worth a try.

Many proponents of barefoot horses claim a long list of advantages to removing shoes. Because there are no scientific studies comparing long-term results of shod versus unshod, much of the discussion on this topic is clouded by exaggeration and biased opinions. It is quite common to find that feet can change from extremely distorted to distortion-free by going from shod to unshod. But exactly the same improvements can be seen when shod feet remain shod in different circumstances such as more frequent shoeing, a different farrier or a different type of trim. The important point is that multiple problems can cause distorted feet and there are multiple solutions to restoring health.

Until you have conducted a thorough balance evaluation, you cannot draw valid conclusions about whether your horse should be barefoot or shod.

Contraction

Contracted feet are too narrow in the heel or throughout the whole foot. A contracted foot looks "shriveled up," particularly in the heel and heel bulb area. There are no objective measurements to determine precisely when a foot is contracted. It is so common for feet to be contracted that slight contraction can be difficult to perceive. Extremely contracted feet are easily identified because the heels are pinched very close together, the frog is usually shrunken, and the whole perimeter of the hoof may be smaller than the perimeter of the coronary band.

The causes of a contracted foot can be neglect, unskilled trimming, or poor shoeing. Let's review a few anatomical facts. Below the sole plane is where the living tissue ends, the caudal part of the hoof is soft tissue only, and the coffin bone is in the front part of the hoof. Contraction occurs when the hoof is overgrown, that is, excess sole and wall horn grow beyond the limits of the healthy hoof.

When excess hoof horn is weak it does not necessarily slough off if the foot is shod. Excess horn can be retained in barefoot horses that do not move enough on hard ground. In this situation, the excess weak horn distorts: it either contracts inwards or squashes outwards, depending on factors such as the horse's posture, weight, and the moisture content of the horn. Because the bone in the front part of the foot helps to keep the wall in a consistent shape, contraction is most easily seen in the back of the foot. Additionally, feet can be too narrow along the entire medial and lateral wall lengths. There is concern that horses shod at a young age, before the bone has reached its adult size and shape, are prone to contracted hooves.

Disadvantages of shoeing popularized in books and articles over the centuries tend to be illogical, basing their argument on cases of poor shoeing or shoes left on far too long. Good shoeing done frequently does not necessarily cause contraction. Contraction and other problems related to shoeing have not been scientifically tested. Farrier experience suggests it is more likely that any hoof distortion, including contraction, is caused by imbalance, neglect, or misapplication of a particular technique. Unless you know for a fact that the shoeing or the barefoot technique is the cause a hoof problem, it does not make sense to blame either of them for hoof distortions.

When shoes are removed from contracted feet, quite often the feet will expand. This does not mean shoeing has caused those feet to become distorted. To demonstrate that shoeing causes contraction, a study would need to track a group of horses shod well by the same farrier over the long-term, and then left barefoot but trimmed consistently by the same farrier over time. Beware of studies that report improvements after shoe removal and attribute them specifically to the shoe removal itself. Any farrier can tell you that a foot that is contracted due to poor shoeing will become larger and healthier when re-shod properly and maintained well.

> **There is concern that horses shod at a young age, before the bone has reached its adult size and shape, are prone to contracted hooves.**

Advantages of Barefoot

A scientific approach to the barefoot balanced hoof has yet to be developed. Currently, anecdotal reports serve as the best evidence. The advantages cited in this discussion are all changes that were observed in horses that were lame or poor movers at the start. All changes were noticed in horses that had shoes removed but nothing else in hoof care changed. The same farrier worked on the horse, the schedule remained the same, and the horse's living situation remained the same.

Sure-footed Movement

Your horse may be more sure-footed in "trappy," rocky terrain. The bare hoof is better able to sense varying ground surfaces, it is better equipped to carry the horse safely and in a more balanced manner over footing that can cause shod horses to slide, stumble, or land too hard. Riders have noticed changes over sections of trail that had caused problems when the horse was shod. Horses that were constantly tripping may become safe to ride again. Horses accustomed to being barefoot have no trouble over rocky terrain when they are going slowly. Some horses, particularly those that have never worn shoes, can trot, canter, and gallop over rocky footing. Riders who pack-trip in the Rocky Mountains can attest to the fact that barefoot horses do well in rough terrain.

> **By being better able to sense the ground with bare feet, the horse is less likely to restrict his own range of motion, which he may have been doing in an effort to make up for his lack of sensory function.**

Improved Range of Motion

Your horse may move with more freedom in his back, shoulder, hock or stifle. Many horses are chronically stiff and tight across their topline and shoulders. There are innumerable possible causes, including tack, rider position, and pain anywhere in the body. One common cause of stiffness and tight muscles is hoof discomfort. Part of the explanation may be simply that a shod horse is less able to feel the ground beneath him. By being better able to sense the ground with bare feet, the horse is less likely to restrict his own range of motion, which he may have been doing in an effort to make up for his lack of sensory function.

This is analogous to the way you would reflexively tighten up your body and take smaller steps when walking on ice or other surfaces that feel perilous. A horse that is not sure how the surface of his feet will react to the ground may have a chronically stiff way of moving in an attempt to feel safe. Some horses attain more swing in their back and stride when barefoot than when they were shod.

Better Quality Hooves

Your horse's feet may stop chipping, flaring, crushing, bruising, contracting, or getting thrush. Outward signs of strong hoof-form are perhaps the most obvious changes that many people notice after keeping feet balanced and unshod. Bruising that sometimes covers large parts of the sole or white line can disappear within weeks or months. Flares may cease to appear when balance is maintained. Often chips and cracks – which can be the foot's way of relieving excess pressure due to imbalance – disappear once the feet are trimmed at appropriate intervals for the individual horse and his growth pattern.

Nailing does not appear to damage strong, thick, healthy wall horn. But feet with healthy wall horn may not need shoes anyway. If a horse with thin wall and sole has sore feet, owners may find that shoes keep the horse sound on hard ground. However, these feet tend to become shell-like and the walls break from nailing. If the horse can afford time off, a barefoot spell may improve the quality of feet. This can render them strong enough for nails again. Additionally, by the time the feet are strong enough for nails, they may be strong enough to stay bare and still perform to the owner's satisfaction.

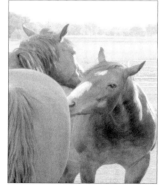

Disadvantages of Barefoot

Scheduling Difficulties

Though it does not entail more work to keep the feet balanced than it does to leave them for months and then take off huge chunks at once, it can be less convenient. The time it takes to trim the hooves is actually longer when there is more time between farrier visits. Trimming often and removing only miniscule amounts at each session probably is equal to or even faster than the conventional approach.

For many horse owners, it is more convenient to pay someone else to take care of their horses' feet. It is easier not to think about it except every few months when you have to go out in the barn and hold horses for the farrier. Even if you want to schedule trimming more frequently, not every farrier is able to visit every few days to one barn to rehabilitate a lame barefoot horse, or even every few weeks to maintain trims on a sound barefoot horse.

Some farriers are happy to have their clients' horses on a four-week schedule or more often for new clients when the feet need very frequent attention to re-establish balance. If your farrier only comes through your area every six or eight or ten weeks, it is unlikely that you can be personally accommodated if you wish to have things done differently. This is one reason many people learn to do some of their own hoof care.

If you can manage the initial investment of time to learn how to rasp, you will ultimately save money and find that it doesn't take much time as you gain competency and your horse's feet get closer to ideal balance.

Loss of Riding Time

A horse may not be sound and rideable during the initial phase of being barefoot. Some horses will be fine right away. Many will be unsound, particularly horses with long-standing hoof weaknesses that have been managed by wearing shoes. One way to get reasonably sound horses rideable faster is to use hoof boots, though it can take some time and patience to find the best hoof boot and the best fit for the types of riding you do. Some people find the boots inconvenient to apply. Others find there are currently no boots on the market that fit well enough in all conditions for their horse to perform in certain sports.

The transition phase for weak feet, while they are slowly healing and regaining their natural strength, is a disadvantageous time for owners. As you can imagine, it is probably time well spent in healing for the horse.

Dealing with Conflicts of Opinion

If you decide to take your horse's hoof care into your own hands, you may find well-meaning friends or neighbors suggesting that you have lost your mind. You may be called arrogant for thinking you can do something that is not your area of expertise.

Trimming is not your expertise and that is exactly why you have a farrier. Not all farriers will tell you the same thing and it can become very confusing. If you've had a farrier say your horse cannot go without shoes, yet you have not actually seen evidence of this because your horse has always been shod, you may want to find a farrier who will be willing to try the barefoot approach.

We all tend to defer to experts somewhat too easily. Farriers do what their training suggests and may not question possible drawbacks of age-old techniques they have become comfortable using. In any particular area the expert is going to know more than you do. For example, your veterinarian is more knowledgeable than you about equine medicine. You find different opinions among practitioners. You can find a practitioner who can direct you toward preventive measures rather than merely ways to manage pain.

Some veterinarians will tell you that laminitic horses never heal fully or even require therapeutic shoeing for the rest of their lives. Just as in human medicine, there are numerous examples of people being told there are no cures, no hope, only medication and a shortened life ahead of them. Sometimes these people have sought alternative medicine only to make a "miraculous," complete recovery.

> **Healing is not usually miraculous. It is an ordinary function of a living being.**

Healing is not usually miraculous. It is an ordinary function of a living being. Provided damage has not progressed beyond a certain point, healing will happen if the impediments are removed, there is an environment for healing, and the horse is capable of healing. If you believe that your horse's present hoof care regime is an impediment to healing, it is up to you to respectfully search for other options.

Things to Discuss with Your Farrier

Shoe Pulling Technique

Having a shoe pulled off can cause trauma to the hoof wall. A diligent farrier will remove the clinches before pulling the shoe. As a time-saving measure, some farriers do not cut clinches, which can result in the inadvertent removal of horn along with the nails at each tug of the shoe. Not only does this damage the hoof horn, but wrenching on the foot can put undue pressure on soft tissues of the leg as well.

Observe your horse's facial and body expression during shoe pulling. Does the horse flinch as clinches are banged off? If so, you might ask your farrier to rasp instead of hammer the clinches off to reduce concussion to the hoof wall. Does the horse have muscles spasms in the body or resist as the farrier pulls the shoe off? If so, ask the farrier to remove each nail one at time with the crease nail pullers. This is not always possible when the nail heads are too worn. Farriers naturally want to save time at each step of the shoeing process, but a good farrier will slow down as needed to keep a horse comfortable and minimize trauma to the foot.

Nails

Using as few nails as possible and making the clinches small minimizes wall damage. Small clinches allow the shoe to come off easily should it get caught in something. Having a shoe that stays on at all costs can cost your horse his own foot. Some farriers put more nails in than the foot really needs, or use oversized nails, because they want extra assurance that the shoe will stay on. It is easier for the farrier to do this than to educate a rider that a shoe coming off is not the worst thing that can happen. Understanding this, you can let your farrier know and he will usually be happy to do a less invasive shoeing on your horse. Most shoes will stay on with fewer nails.

There are options to nailing. A variety of materials are now available for creating pour-on adhesive shoes. There are also glues for attaching steel or plastic shoes to the hoof. Several hoof boot companies are selling horse sneakers, moccasins, and other equine foot wear. Ask your farrier about these alternatives if your thin-walled horse needs hoof protection.

Shoe Shape

When the toe of the shoe follows the natural outline of the hoof, the shoe will preserve the shape of the hoof. Front feet are round because this is the most functional shape to assist the major weight bearing and support. The round hoof allows the foot to easily break over laterally when the horse needs to move sideways. Hind feet are slightly pointy because this is the most functional shape to allow the horse to pivot, and to permit the toe to dig in slightly so the horse can use the hind end for propulsion.

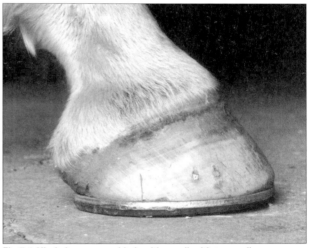

Fig 5.1 Hind shoe secured in healthy wall with two nails on the medial side (the lateral side had three nails).

There are manufactured shoes that come pre-shaped in front and hind patterns. There are unshaped generic pattern shoes that cost less and are designed to be shaped by the farrier. Some farriers, to save time and money, purchase the unshaped shoes and nail them on to the feet regardless of the horse's hoof shape. A basic principle of shoeing is that over time, feet attain the shape of the steel. Horse feet are not naturally oblong shaped. If shod this way for long enough, they do become this shape. So if a farrier says "I'm just shoeing to his foot shape", you might wonder if at some point in the past

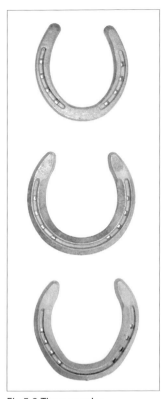

Fig 5.2 Three popular pre-made (keg) shoes. Top, unshaped shoe. Middle, front shape. Bottom, hind shape.

a farrier played a part in creating that foot shape! If those elongated "compromise pattern" feet are trimmed and shod differently, they can regain their natural shape.

There are farriers who like square toes because they say it can help keep the feet traveling straight. Most horses are not perfectly conformed. Being forced to break over in the middle of the foot can overload other structures in the limb. Your farrier may tell you the square toe moves the breakover point back. The breakover point can also be moved back by rolling or "rockering," rather than squaring the toe.

Square toes may have a place on certain horses; but ask for an explanation from your farrier before doing it. Many farriers believe that the altered shape of squaring the toe reduces the horse's ability to use his feet as they were intended. If your farrier can explain why your horse needs this special shape, then perhaps the horse does. Do not accept square toes just because that is the "trademark" look of a particular farrier.

Shoe Size

Placing a sufficiently large shoe with plenty of heel support on the hoof can minimize contraction and heel bruising. Most horses move better in shoes that are set full with branches supporting the heels, tightly fit shoes are usually only needed if the horse otherwise cannot keep shoes on, or interferes. The term "set full" refers to a shoe that is placed so you can see steel sticking out beyond the foot in the quarters and heels.

A disconcertingly large percentage of farriers still use a small shoe, shod tight and short at the heels. They may be doing it because they believe it best, or because they lack the skill to set a shoe full. Many trainers ask for a small shoe because they *assume* a larger one won't stay in place. The assumption, however, is often not borne out once you actually try the larger size. Give your horse the benefit of the doubt and experiment at least once with shoes set full.

For discussion about stock thickness, width and other shoeing considerations it is helpful to read a farrier textbook, such as Butler's *Principles of Horseshoeing II*. Since this is probably the book your farrier read at shoeing school, it will be useful for you to know the basics.

Clips

Clips are small triangular tabs along the edge of the shoe that help to secure shoe fit. Clips can be hand-forged on steel shoes by a skilled farrier, or factory-made shoes can be purchased pre-clipped. Hand-forged clips can be placed anywhere the foot needs them, and are particularly advantageous if a foot has much broken out wall where nails cannot be placed. Factory-made shoes come in two standard clip arrangements: toe clips or side clips. Traditionally, toe clips were popular on front feet and side clips popular on hind feet. It is common today to see side clips on all four feet.

If your horse tends to lose shoes easily, clips might help. There are inherent risks with a clipped shoe. If wrenched partially off, it may shift on the foot and cause a puncture wound in the sole or frog. Also, lost shoes with clips are hazardous to other horses out in the pasture.

A skilled farrier can make a clip that fits the angle of the wall perfectly and needs no traumatic banging to get them in place. Concerns about the possible risks to the outer hoof wall come more from observation of poorly set clips than any inherent problem with clips. Ask your farrier about the benefits and risks of using clips. Many farriers like clips because they help to take shearing stress off of the nails and help to hold shoes in place on horses that tend to twist their feet upon landing. Clips are often used for hooves that have weak walls and do not hold nails well.

Unless they fit well, clips must be banged hard with a hammer. Once hammered in, a clip permanently compresses hoof wall that is directly attached to the laminae. In some horses this can cause discomfort from excess pressure. Avoiding clips reduces possible trauma to the hoof wall and internal structures. The foot is made to take a pounding from the ground surface where nails are driven, but the foot is not well equipped to take a blow from the front and side where clips are placed. Over time, the hammering in of clips can stress the inside of the foot more than hammering in nails.

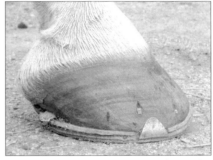

Fig 5.3 Clips can help stabilize the shoe and reduce stress of the nails. The clipped shoe in this photo required fewer nails and the pad remained secure throughout the shoeing period.

Toe clips, according to some farriers, are potentially more detrimental than side clips because in order to apply a toe clip, the shoe must be set in front of the toe wall and this often sets the breakover point too far forward. This criticism of toe clips is valid on long-toed horses that need a shoe set flush with or behind the toe edge of the hoof wall. Toe clips are fine and possibly even advantageous on a short-toed horse that might benefit from a slightly longer toe.

Padding

Your farrier will be able to explain the advantages and disadvantages of using pads. Common reasons for using pads include supporting the sole, providing shock absorption, and changing the angle of the hoof by using a wedge.

Horse owners commonly assume that pads are for foot-sore horses. This is true in limited cases. For example, when the coffin bone is dropped, some horses benefit from having a pad between the foot and the shoe. In many cases, a horse is foot-sore on hard roads due to something other than sole soreness.

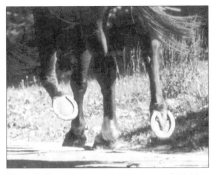

Fig 5.4 Some horses are more comfortable wearing pads on gravel roads.

Quite often owners will request pads on foot-sore horse and then find that it makes no difference. In these cases, the foot soreness may be due to imbalance, and padding has no effect on that.

A heavy horse or one with soft soles may suffer from dropped soles over the long term. Pads with packing and added frog support can help prevent dropping. However, the foot can sometimes become too damp underneath the pad, leading to additional frog and sole softening and sometimes thrush. When a horse works on soft ground, the turf or dirt will fill in the foot and support the sole so no pad is needed. You might find that alternating between pads for one shoeing and open shoes the next is a good compromise for your horse.

For shock absorption, there are a variety of materials although little research exists to substantiate claims about whether or not significant energy dissipation is achieved.

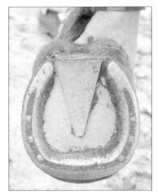

Fig 5.5 To support or possibly prevent dropped soles, additional frog support material fills in space between shoe edge and ground.

Using a pad to wedge a foot is controversial. Most farriers agree that using a heel wedge results in a degree of crushed horn at the heels. There is some research on the use of wedges but there is no agreement on how farriers ought to weigh the trade-offs of correcting a broken back hoof pastern axis versus causing crushed heel horn. You and your farrier must discuss your horse's specific case to decide if it is worth trying wedge pads.

Shoe Material

Most horseshoes are made of steel, which is still the most economical and versatile material available. Aluminum is a popular alternative for horses that may benefit from a more lightweight shoe. Unfortunately, there are several disadvantages to aluminum. When aluminum is heated, its properties change and it is difficult for farriers to do forge work on aluminum.

Once heated, the metal is weaker. Aluminum is a poor choice for hard roads: it is softer than steel and thus wears very quickly. For a horse working on soft, non-abrasive ground, such as grass, aluminum could be a good shoe material.

There are many varieties of plastic or polyurethane shoes. Each shoe type has advantages and disadvantages regarding ease of use, durability, and versatility. Most are considerably more expensive than either steel or aluminum. Some specialized shoes require considerable farrier experience to ensure successful application. If you wish to try a new type of shoe, find a farrier who has put them on other horses. Ask if your horse would be a good candidate for the shoes.

Shoeing Schedule

Having a frequent shoeing schedule reduces hoof distortion and balance problems that grow worse over time. Since many shod feet tend to grow slowly, farriers are hesitant to schedule shoeing appointments too close together because they can run out of places to put nails. If you need to keep the horse shod year round, consider a few times when he can be barefoot for a week or two between shoeing. You may find that this will result in enough growth to re-shoe more easily.

Consider shoeing the front feet only. This allows the hind feet to have all the benefits of bare feet and for many horses, hinds do not get sore even in the rockiest terrain. Some farriers feel that a horse should either be shod all around or be barefoot all around and that shoeing half the horse will result in balance problems. Many horses have been shod on the front feet only without any detectable problems. There are no studies to suggest that this is a problem.

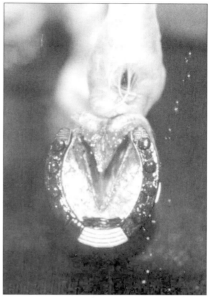

Fig 5.6 Special shock absorbing shoe with changeable synthetic inserts for different traction needs, this Slypner Athletic Sport Shoe works well for certain horses.

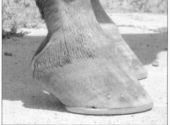 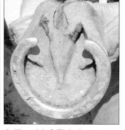

Fig 5.7a, 5.7b Do your horse's feet look like this? This horse is blessed with good hoof mass and strong horn which keep these feet looking strong with no toe wall distortion, no crushed heels, and no chipped wall in the area of the nail holes despite having eight nails in each foot. The long toe and long heel mean the feet are off balance. If neglected for months, even feet that looked good on the day they were shod can end up looking like this. Sometimes feet look like this shortly after being shod if hooves were not properly trimmed before shoes were applied.

Hoof Preparation

How to trim for shoeing is an ongoing area of controversy in farrier circles. Ask your farrier to explain the trim method and to tell you why certain parts are taken out with the

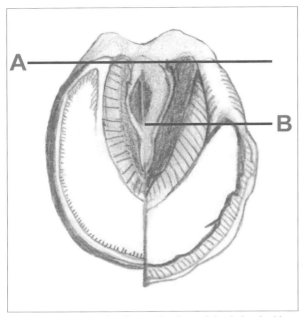

Fig 5.8 Line A depicts hoof properly trimmed: heels level with base of frog. Line B on untrimmed half shows heels too far forward. Also notice, the untrimmed side has a stretched white line.

knife and other parts are left alone. From the information you have gained from this book, clinics, other texts or websites, you will be better equipped to have a productive discussion with your farrier.

Dealing with Pain

Considering the many dimensions of whole horse health, shoeing can be beneficial. For example, a horse that is uncomfortable and therefore not ride-able for long periods of time may become emotionally despondent. Coupled with the unhappiness of the horse owner who cannot ride, the relationship between horse and human may suffer. Shoeing a horse that feels anxious or sad when not working can relieve pain and allow him to perform his job again. This can provide emotional benefits that outweigh any temporary reduction of healing inside the hoof. A horse that is uncomfortable even in his own pasture when left barefoot may need shoes so that he can move around comfortably. If he can be ridden too, this will bring cardiovascular and muscular benefits, important components of whole horse healing even if they temporarily slow hoof growth or reduce progress in laminar regeneration.

It is challenging for us to think from the horse's point of view but we must endeavor to consider things from different perspectives. If a horse is in pain for a long period of time and cannot happily romp around his own pasture or play with pasture-mates, he will suffer in more ways than we may realize.

Sometimes pain is an unavoidable part of healing and to block it out is to invite more troublesome consequences in the future. Only you can decide how long the pain is "good," in the sense that it is allowing the hoof to heal, and when the diminishing returns of chronic pain must be considered. Movement is important, but damaged feet need controlled, slow movement. This is one reason giving a painkiller can cause more problems than it solves. If a horse feels good and runs around on fragile feet, the result can be additional traumatic damage. On the other hand if a barefoot horse is unable to move because his feet hurt, the benefits of putting on shoes or giving him medication may outweigh the harms. Some horses are simply too sore when barefoot, even in boots, to move around on hard ground. If this is the only type of surface you have, then short of covering your turnout area in artificial turf or rubber mats, there are no good options.

There is no way to know for sure at what point any potential benefits of returning the horse to light work through shoeing or administering painkillers might outweigh the risks. Your intuition and knowledge of your horse's personality must guide you, along with the analyses and suggestions from your farrier, veterinarian and other equine health practitioners.

Chapter highlights

- Balance is the essential requirement regardless of shoeing or barefoot. Once balance is achieved, it can be maintained with frequent farrier appointments.
- Possible advantages of barefoot hoof care include improved hoof quality, soundness, range of motion and sure-footedness over varied terrain.
- If your horse works on hard or abrasive terrain, shoes may be necessary if the horse wears the feet faster than they can re-grow.
- If you decide your horse requires shoeing, discuss the shoe specifications with your farrier to be sure your horse gets what is needed in terms of shoe size, shape, padding, clips and nailing.
- Be attentive to signs of pain. Breaking a cycle of pain is important in order for a horse to heal. Some horses need shoes to break the pain cycle; others need to be barefoot.

Recommended Reading

Horse Owner's Guide to Natural Hoof Care, Jaime Jackson
Making Natural Hoof Care Work for You, Pete Ramey

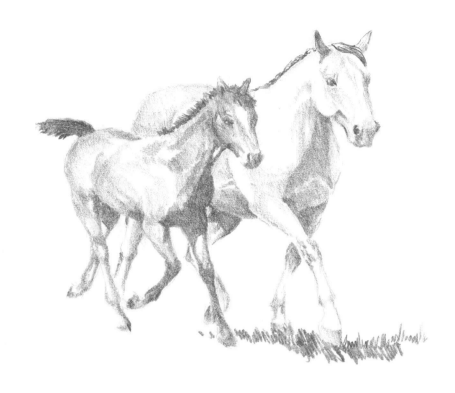

And indeed, a horse who bears himself proudly is a thing of such beauty and astonishment that he attracts the eyes of all beholders; no one will tire of looking at him as long as he will display himself in his splendor.

— Xenophon

chapter six

Laminitis and Navicular

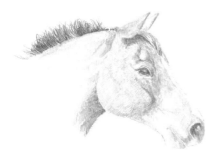

- **The Multiple Causes of Laminitis**
- **Laminitis is Preventable and Curable**
- **Navicular Syndrome is a Manageable Condition**
- **Maintaining Balance Reduces the Risk of Hoof Disease**

Imagine a small covered bridge on a country road. A posted warning sign reads "Weight Limit 10 Tons." A local contractor regularly drives his eighteen-ton dump truck over this stoutly built structure. It didn't collapse the first time he did it, and it didn't collapse the fiftieth time he crossed in the overweight truck, so you're pretty sure that when you cross it in your nine-ton truck and loaded hay wagon, it will hold you just fine. Lucky for you the river is not too far down or too deep, because with shocking suddenness, the bridge gives way and you find yourself landing in the cold water with a mighty splash. As you scramble out of the river, you wonder "why me and why now?"

The answer is simple. Every time the bridge was overstressed, its timbers and joints were consistently weakened and the bridge shifted minutely on its foundation. As the overloading continued, the damage and misalignment grew, causing more of the weight to be supported by the weakened structure. When you arrived with your hay truck, your load was the "last straw" to cross that bridge.

Owners whose horses are afflicted by laminitis and navicular usually feel a similar sense of surprise and shock if their horse suffers from these debilitating ailments. Laminitis and navicular syndrome are the two main hoof disorders that have the potential for crippling horses. This chapter explains what laminitis and navicular are, what you can do to reduce the risks related to these ailments, and how to respond if they occur.

Horse people often consider laminitis and navicular to be equine analogues to feared human ailments, like heart disease or cancer. Exact causes and mechanisms of these complex human diseases remain unknown, but certain preventive measures can be taken. We also know that multiple factors, such as diet, lifestyle, toxin exposure, and genetics act in concert to influence one's susceptibility profile. This holds true for human and equine alike.

Much remains unanswered about these disease processes. In general, doing "everything right" reduces the chances of disease. Even when few identifiable risk factors appear to exist, horses still get laminitis or navicular. Genetic predisposition almost certainly plays a role. There are horses that seem prone to hoof problems despite good care, and others stay strong and sound despite poor hoof care.

While these two disorders have the potential for significant harm, the actions you take have the potential to reverse injury and maintain soundness. Armed with knowledge, you can turn fear into determination and optimism.

Laminitis

Laminitis is presented first in this chapter because it is a time-critical emergency. If you are not sure whether lameness is due to laminitis or navicular, it is safe to begin emergency treatment for laminitis. If it turns out your horse has navicular or some other cause of lameness, the treatment for laminitis may not be needed, but it is unlikely to cause harm. On the other hand, if your horse is suffering from laminitis, failure to treat it immediately may result in things going critically wrong within a short period of time.

What is laminitis?

The literal, medical definition of laminitis is inflammation of the laminae. The more commonly recognized definition is "failure of the laminar bond," according to noted Australian researcher and veterinarian, Dr. Chris Pollitt, BVSc, PhD. The word "failure" is misleading because it sounds ominous. You might think of catastrophic breakdown when you hear the term failure. The breakdown of the bond can range from long-term, mild and clinically undetectable to severe and crippling within a matter of hours or days. A more neutral way to explain laminitis is to call it dysfunction or a defect in some or all of the laminae. Mild dysfunction is not too frightening. Severe dysfunction may well lead to widespread failure if all or most of the laminar bond breaks down.

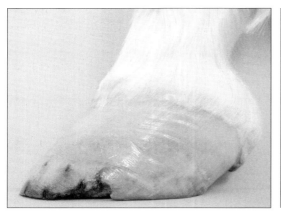 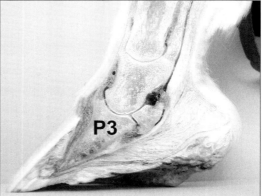

Fig 6.1a and 6.1b This foundered hoof specimen is seen from two views. Looking at the outer hoof wall, notice the characteristic rings diverging at the heel, upward bulge in the hairline at the quarter, long underrun heel, and long toe. Looking inside this hoof, notice the loss of parallel relationship between dorsal hoof wall and coffin bone (P3).

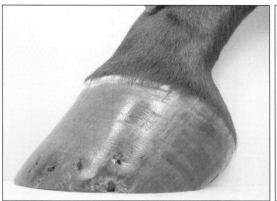 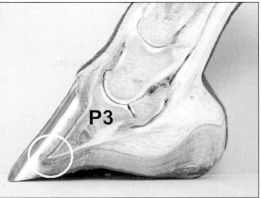

Fig 6.2a and 6.2b Normal bone alignment, no outward signs of laminitis. The dorsal hoof wall and P3 are parallel; P3 is high in the hoof capsule; and there is ample sole depth. One indication that this foot has not been ideally balanced is the small lip of bone at the tip of P3. This "ski-tip" shape to the bone tends to remain asymptomatic in horses with good sole depth. But, it is an indicator that the foot needs to be rebalanced or the horse may eventually become lame.

The laminae secure the coffin bone (P3) to the hoof wall. An analogy describing this bond is that of super strong Velcro. Unlike Velcro, the laminar bond is not designed to come apart. Studies conducted in Pollitt's lab have documented many of the mechanisms of laminitis. An interesting experiment was done on the mechanical properties of the laminar junction using fresh cadaver feet. Investigators tested the strength of the laminar bond to see how much force it would take to rip the tissues apart from the wall. In the laminitic feet, they were able to pull apart tissues at the epidermal-dermal junction where the sensitive and insensitive laminae are interwoven.

Investigators found that in healthy feet the bond between hoof wall and coffin bone could not be broken. Instead of the tissue ripping at the dermal-epidermal junction, in healthy feet it actually broke off right from the bone. This tells us something about a healthy horse foot. It is indestructible as far as the dermal-epidermal junction goes. Something must be terribly wrong to cause the horse's foot to fall apart.

The term "founder" is often used interchangeably with laminitis. However, the two terms are clinically distinct. Laminitis is quite common. When mild, it tends to be self-limiting. Even if severe, many cases of laminitis are correctable with changes in hoof care, diet and/or the use of anti-inflammatory drugs.

Founder, a more serious condition, refers to movement of the coffin bone away from its normal position within the hoof capsule due to the failure of laminar attachments. The coffin bone may rotate in any direction, but most commonly the distal tip rotates down toward the sole, putting pressure against the sole in front of the frog. The coffin bone may also displace distally all at once. In other words, without rotating, it may sink to the bottom of the foot and place pressure on the whole sole. Termed "sinking founder," this form of founder happens when all the laminar attachments fail at once.

The front feet are more prone to founder. When it appears in all four feet, it is usually worse in the front. This is probably because the front feet carry a greater proportion of the horse's body weight. But be aware that horses may founder only in the hind feet, or even in just one hind foot. If laminitis is suspected, or founder detected, you need to be on the lookout for it in all of the feet.

Laminitis and founder may appear to happen simultaneously. Given that founder is caused by dysfunction of the laminae, and that healthy laminae do not fail, we assume that if a horse has foundered, it was preceded by laminitis.

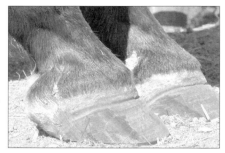

Fig 6.3 Front feet with deep founder ridges. This photo was taken 6 weeks after diagnosis. Regular trimming has balanced the feet so there are no other outward signs of laminitis.

Causes and Mechanisms of Laminitis

The laminar junction is a critical structural component of the hoof. It joins the coffin bone to the hoof wall while allowing the natural flexion and expansion of the hoof. This structure is amazingly strong and flexible. When stresses are placed on the laminae in correct alignment, the laminae are more likely to remain healthy.

Laminitis research today is a fast-moving field. Dr. Chris Pollitt continues to discover new clinically important information. Another leading-edge laminitis researcher is David Hood, DVM, PhD, of The Hoof Project research lab. Hood's lab developed a technique for collecting laminar junction tissue samples from live horses. This development allowed Hood and his team of investigators to experimentally induce laminitis, study sections of these horses' feet under the microscope, and treat the horses for full return to soundness. This was a major advance; it meant horses need not be killed for the sake of the scientific process. It also enhanced the investigation of early signs of laminar compromise that appear prior to the onset of clinical signs.

Regardless of the research controversy and existing gaps in scientific understanding, you still have to take charge of your horse's fate. You must be able to recognize risk factors and warning signs, be empowered to design a sound prevention plan, and be ready to respond to an emergency.

Much of the fear and concern surrounding laminitis is because there is little agreement in the research literature on its causes and treatments. While researchers agree that laminitis is correlated with improper hoof loading and/or altered blood flow within the hoof, it is not yet known if vascular changes are the cause or the consequence of other malfunctions.

Current research focusing on the complex and mysterious nature of metabolic processes in laminitis may eventually yield breakthroughs in prevention and treatment.

While acknowledging the importance of metabolic issues, we cannot overlook a critical but underemphasized factor in most hoof disorders: mechanical stress may cause or contribute to laminitic failure. Hence, hoof balance may be a key component in the prevention and treatment of laminitis.

In the hoof, overstress is rarely caused by too much weight alone, but by having weight improperly supported due to unbalanced hooves. Toes or heels that are too long can put laminae under excessive shear stress. Laminae can be compressed and bruised by lateral misalignment or under-run heels. In a healthy well-balanced foot, the hoof wall shares the load with other structures. Part of the sole, bar and frog also act to support weight. When the horse's weight is being supported by the hoof wall alone, the coffin bone is effectively hanging from the laminae, again causing critical shear stress. Once this damage begins, it weakens the structure and places increased stress on the remaining laminae. Additionally, the internal damage is likely to cause inflammation and swelling, leading to impaired circulation and metabolic function. At some point, the combination of mechanical and metabolic dysfunction causes enough damage to manifest as laminitis. Once this occurs, in order to affect a recovery, you must address both the mechanical and metabolic issues.

Metabolism-based Theories

To date, the two leading metabolism-based theories on laminitis can be summarized as the vascular theory and the enzymatic theory. The vascular theory states that reduced blood flow to the laminae can result in cell death leading to the weakening of the laminar bond. The enzymatic theory states that initially blood flow remains normal, but toxic trigger factors cause an enzymatic malfunction in laminar cells resulting in destruction of the bond. In principle these theories are not mutually exclusive, yet there is fierce debate over the relative importance of each process. Because the research studies differ in their methodology and terminology, it is not possible to make direct comparisons of the competing theories.

While the research debates rage, the historical evidence allows us to recognize that any of the following conditions can serve as contributing factors to laminitis: carbohydrate overload, obesity, pregnancy, medical

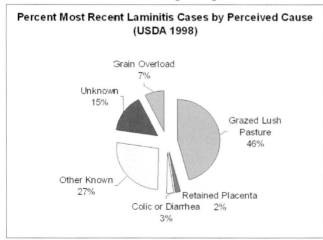

Fig 6.4 Statistics indicate that over half of all laminitis cases are attributed to feed management problems.

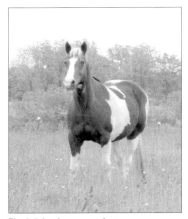

Fig 6.5 Lush pasture is a common factor in laminitis.

conditions, and abnormal stress. No single risk factor can predict whether your horse will become laminitic. There are plenty of horses that are theoretically at risk, but the majority of them do not get laminitis. For instance, pregnancy is a known risk factor, but most brood mares do not have laminitis.

According to the US Department of Agriculture's National Animal Health Monitoring System, a large survey study of data from over 28,000 horses across the country, only 2.1% were reported to have laminitis, either chronic or acute, during 1998-1999 when the study was conducted. This tells us that most horses do not become laminitic. Of horses that are reported lame, laminitis is likely to be the cause in up to 40% of the cases. Though this book focuses only on the hoof, be aware that limb and joint problems account for up to 50% of equine lameness, according to the USDA study.

A scientific understanding does not yet exist for many of the risk factors that appear to contribute to laminitis. Consider each factor in turn to appreciate possible reasons why these are risks.

Overeating is generally considered the prime cause of laminitis. The mechanism appears to be the following sequence of events. A large dose of rapidly fermentable carbohydrate alters the normal intestinal pH. The pH change disrupts the normal microbial population, causing large numbers of "friendly bacteria" to die. The irritated intestinal lining becomes inflamed and leaky. Toxins make their way into the blood stream and eventually reach the feet. Toxic trigger factors then cause vascular changes and/or disrupt normal enzymatic processes in the laminae, leading to laminar bond weakening and destruction.

Carbohydrate overload is the most commonly used experimental method to induce laminitis. It is usually not a foray into the grain room that you have to be cautious of. According to the above-mentioned USDA study the perceived cause of almost half (45.6%) of all laminitis is grazing in "lush pasture" with grain overload only comprising approximately 7% of cases. The study concluded that "proper grazing and feed management could prevent approximately one-half of laminitis cases."

Obesity may be associated with carbohydrate overload, not in the acute sense like the experimental model, but in a gradual fashion. A

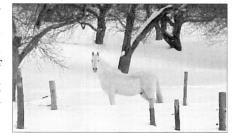

Fig 6.6 Horses can become laminitic even in the winter. Grain overload and/or reduced water intake are common contributing laminitis factors during the winter.

horse that consumes more calories than it needs may have sub-clinical carbohydrate overload, increasing the risk that an added factor might cause overt laminitis. Additionally, obesity means the horse might simply carry too much weight on its feet. The mechanical stress placed on laminae weakened by carbohydrate metabolism dysfunction can accelerate laminitic degeneration. Often such horses have appeared sound for some time, and it is not obvious to a casual observer why it "suddenly" became laminitic. If obesity is associated with endocrine dysfunction such as a thyroid or pituitary problem, the horse may have an even higher risk of laminitis.

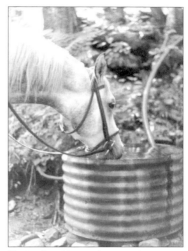

Fig 6.7 Provide ample water in the winter. Water heaters may be needed.

Several factors occur simultaneously that may explain why certain mares become laminitic during pregnancy. Unfortunately, brood mares are often not given high priority for trimming. Combine this with the increase in body weight during gestation. Long and unbalanced feet can become mechanically unstable. Then add hormonally related physiological changes during pregnancy. All of these factors can lead to dysfunction of the laminitic bond.

During pregnancy, there is a general condition of immune suppression, which is a normal physiological mechanism so that the mare's body does not reject the fetus. In this state of immune suppression, the mare herself is at greater risk of several potential laminitis trigger factors including allergies.

Another change during pregnancy is a general relaxing of elastic connective tissue. This may affect the laminar junction causing it to stretch and weaken. A final reproductive risk that is known to cause laminitis is a retained placenta. The mechanism in this case, as with some other metabolic causes, is that circulation of toxins damages the cells at the laminar junction.

Other medical conditions such as colic, and colic surgery, and infectious diseases such as Potomac Horse Fever are also common precursors to laminitis. A 2003 study from Texas A&M University found that horses with chronic laminitis had higher immune reactivity to injected allergens than non-laminitic horses. This study was not designed to test a cause and effect relationship between laminitis and allergic conditions, but researchers did conclude that horses known to be laminitic might be more prone to hypersensitivity reactions such as an allergic reaction to vaccination.

Horses with allergic conditions, including common problems such as heaves or skin allergies, might be more prone to laminitis, although no studies have yet examined if laminitis is a cause or result of immune hyper-reactivity.

Abnormal physiological stress comes to horses from a broad array of activities and situations in which we routinely place them. Shipping, competing, training, illness, vaccinating, deworming, and medicating: these can all be trigger factors for laminitis. The mechanisms may include immune mediated reactions, toxins from gut flora disturbances or external sources, and body-wide inflammatory responses that eventually affect the hoof circulation.

A potential cofactor in all of the triggers mentioned is off-balance feet. When feet are neglected they can become too long, lopsided, flared, or cracked. The laminae inside those feet are being stretched, stressed or bent. Thus, neglect can lead to the foot experiencing unnatural force. Some of the many tiny capillaries vital to effective circulation may be compressed, reducing their function. Laminae can respond and adapt to less than ideal forces. Laminae can proliferate as well as undergo shape changes. But at some point they give way and can no longer do their job. This horse will then be at higher risk for laminitis.

How is Laminitis Diagnosed?

Clinical indicators are generally used to diagnose laminitis, from mild to severe. X-rays will always reveal founder by showing the rotation of P3 or the hoof capsule, but since laminitis does not always progress to founder, x-rays may be of limited use in diagnosing laminitis alone. The horse's medical history is very important because certain factors such as diet, exercise, drug use, and concurrent or previous existence of other conditions are all possible risk factors for laminitis.

X-Rays

When your horse needs a foot x-ray, you can help by having the foot marked prior to the veterinarian's arrival. It is important to mark the feet so that the relationship between the hoof capsule and the bones can be clearly identified. Research on these x-ray parameters was first published in Robert Linford's 1987 doctorate dissertation and was based on studies of racing thoroughbreds. There have been no studies establishing whether or to what extent the parameters differ across the horse population, so this is still an inexact science. The precise number of millimeters for normal ranges is not yet known. Interpretation of your horse's x-rays may vary from one veterinarian to another. Over the past 15 years, practitioners specializing in equine podiatry, such as Dr. Ric Redden in Kentucky, or Dr. Barbara Page in Colorado, have conducted clinical research to clarify and refine diagnostic x-ray techniques for the horse's hoof.

For the first marker, place a thin wire starting exactly at the hairline and running down along the dorsal wall. You can tape this right to the wall. The second marker is a thumbtack you place directly into the tip of the frog. See the accompanying illustrations and the captions explaining of few things the veterinarian will check including depth of

How Do You Know If Your Horse is Laminitic?

Keep in mind the acknowledged causes and contributors to laminitis (i.e., excess weight, overeating, off-balance feet, and metabolic stress) as you review the list of clinical signs.

Clinical Signs of Laminitis:
Early signs:
- Reluctance to move freely
- Blood stain visible in the white line
- Pulse and respiration may be elevated due to pain
- When moving, prefers to canter rather than trot if given a choice
- Feet are off balance, may have long toes, high heels, or both
- Moves forward soundly but takes slightly shorter than normal strides
- Sound on soft terrain but may limp or stumble on hard or rocky ground
- Sole bruising and a stretched white line (note: in some horses by the time you see this they have been compromised for quite some time).

Late signs:
- Lies down
- Standing, but will not move
- Bounding digital pulse
- Sole hot to the touch
- White line stretched
- Will not allow you to pick up a foot
- Stops eating
- Sole bruise in the shape of the coffin bone
- Shifting weight from foot to foot in front (swaying from side to side)
- Standing with front legs stretched out, back arched, trying to lean back to get weight off toes
- When asked to turn in a tight area like in a stall or narrow barn aisle the horse rocks backward onto haunches, lifts head up and lurches around because it hurts to turn the feet.

A horse standing with his front legs extended, back arched, and trying to lean back is the most common indicator of late-stage laminar degeneration. There may be other reasons a horse would stand this way but almost invariably it means the horse has foundered. All of the other signs listed need to be evaluated in context. No single indicator would be diagnostic for laminitis. Usually several of these signs will appear together or appear over the course of a few days.

Chronic laminitic feet may have characteristic rings on the hoof wall that are wider apart at the heels than at the toe. This is due to slower growth at the toe than the heel, which seems to be due to reduced blood supply to the front of the foot. A foot with this growth ring pattern may have been left too long in between farrier visits or been balanced incorrectly so that heel growth exceeded toe growth.

What to Do If You Suspect Laminitis

Gene Ovnicek's pioneering work has led to today's standard emergency treatment for laminitic horses. He found that for severely laminitic horses, the use of Styrofoam foot padding can save a horse's life and set it on the road to full recovery. Following Ovnicek's innovative work, hoof care practitioners the world over have found that supporting the sole is central to most therapeutic approaches. Ovnicek found that horses in too much pain to be shod were best assisted with foam padding. In Ovnicek's treatment system, therapeutic shoes may be nailed on after a horse has become stabilized and pain free when wearing foam. This could be a matter or days, weeks, or even months in some cases.

There are other treatment plans in which shoes are never nailed on at all. Controversy exists over the best way to manage either severe or mild chronic laminitis. You will need to fully discuss options with your veterinarian and farrier. The key point is that for emergency treatment of laminitis, you should apply foam padding immediately. See the resource section of this book for information on Ovnicek's foam emergency kits as well as other ideas for foot padding.

You can safely begin the foam support therapy before the veterinarian and farrier arrive. In addition to foam padding, hosing or soaking the feet in cold water is also indicated to reduce inflammation. Both of these therapies, applying foam and soaking in cold water, usually reduce pain in a horse already showing signs.

Since damage occurs before the horse shows lameness, it is wise to provide preemptive treatment. You can initiate hydrotherapy and/or foam padding after a hard competition, during illness (particularly one with a fever), or after colic surgery.

While it is important to take these steps right away, they are not a substitute for professional help. You need a veterinarian to take x-rays, make a diagnosis, and assist you and the farrier with the best treatment plan.

Prevention and Treatment

The best prevention is regular hoof care to maintain balance, an appropriate diet, and an exercise routine to maintain appropriate body condition. Any time your horse experiences a stressful event it is wise to monitor closely for subtle signs of foot pain. The stress can be something as simple as routine vaccination, de-worming, or being worked hard when the horse is not physically fit. When the horse is ill, has a fever, or stops eating – whether from colic, infectious disease or traumatic injury anywhere on the body – you need to be alert for possible laminitis. Another common cause is an injury to one leg, causing the horse to overload the other side (the stronger leg), resulting in what is termed "support limb laminitis." Any kind of joint, ligament or tendon injury is liable to result in support limb complications.

Research has shown that by the time you see obvious clinical signs, significant laminar damage has already occurred. This means you must be proactive and very observant to catch it early. A vet may declare a horse sound because there is no obvious limp. If your horse moves more tentatively than normal, only you will know. Some vets are not familiar with early signs of laminitis because they are only called out to treat emergencies. It is up to you, the guardian of your horse's health, to recognize early signs.

X-rays are usually used to confirm a clinical diagnosis of founder. Yet x-rays can be deceptive, because they only mark a single point in time. If the x-ray shows the bone out of place, treatment is clearly needed immediately. However a "good" x-ray does not mean you are in the clear. The bone could move at any time if the horse is showing clinical signs. Many horses are declared "not foundered" based on x-rays and yet the farrier can see subtle signs in the foot. To make things more complicated, some horses do not show clinical signs until an enormous amount of damage has accumulated. A horse may look fine and the vet will tell you no x-rays are needed. If you have any concern, get x-rays.

Some veterinarians do not distinguish between laminitis and founder. They may look only for grave signs of founder, and dismiss any indication of mild inflammation in the foot as insignificant. *Any* pain at all in the foot is significant. Though your horse may be stoic, he is never happy to be in pain. It is your obligation to respond immediately.

Because laminitis is known to be a "whole horse disorder," a holistic approach works well to identify and correct the root cause. Proper nutrition is an essential component in laminitis prevention and treatment. The role of gastrointestinal health is always central to holistic approaches.

Navicular Syndrome

Navicular syndrome, in its most general sense, involves pain in the back part of the foot in or near the navicular bone. The definition and diagnosis of navicular syndrome is controversial. Many clinicians have found that navicular syndrome involves damage and inflammation either to the navicular bone, navicular bursa, or deep digital flexor tendon in the navicular area. Some believe that the pain originates elsewhere in the foot, and that pain specific to the navicular area is secondary to another insult.

The lameness associated with navicular syndrome tends to be of slow onset and does not always appear related to the work the horse was doing. In fact, some horses develop navicular before beginning serious training. It usually shows up intermittently, and over time becomes progressively more severe. Unlike laminitis, navicular is not an emergency.

Navicular is most commonly seen in the front feet, though it can occur in the hind feet. It is usually more severe in one front foot but tends to occur in both. While a horse with navicular shows some of the same signs as mild laminitis, such as reluctance to move forward freely or reluctance to hold a foot up, navicular has its own distinct signs.

Clinical Signs of Navicular:
- Tripping, stumbling
- Prefers to trot rather than canter
- Standing with one foot pointed forward
- One foot is smaller with steep, upright heels
- Reluctance to swing the leg freely forward, "flat" mover, short stride
- May have concurrent signs of mild laminitis, particularly in the foot that shows less navicular pain (i.e., support limb laminitis).

To date, there is no experimental model for understanding navicular and no way to induce it in research horses. Therefore, tracking causes and mechanisms of navicular is an even greater research challenge than it is for laminitis. Currently, navicular is considered by conventional veterinary medicine to be incurable. Unlike laminitis, it does not appear to be related to metabolic problems, dietary factors, or concurrent disease processes.

Diagnosing Navicular

There is wide disagreement about the value of common navicular diagnostic tests including x-rays, hoof testers and nerve blocks. With traditional diagnostic tools yielding little information, practitioners attempt to diagnose the problem by the horse's response to therapies such as corrective shoeing and pharmacological approaches like vasodilators or bone remodeling drugs. In fact, the diagnosis of navicular has become so controversial that some clinicians feel the term is meaningless. Focus on the generalized heel pain rather than the navicular area specifically leads many veterinarians to use the terms "palmar hoof syndrome" or "caudal hoof syndrome" or "caudal heel syndrome." Recall from Chapter 2 that palmar refers to the back half of the horse's foot and is used interchangeably with caudal.

If your horse has been diagnosed with heel pain, what does this mean? What can you do about it? Is it an incurable degenerative condition? Take heart, there is anecdotal evidence that some cases of heel pain are reversible. Despite our lack of scientific understanding, there are things you can do that may prevent as well as treat

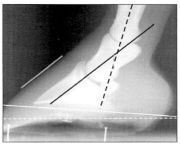
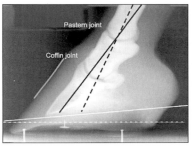

Fig 6.13 These two x-rays are front feet of an 8 year old Quarter Horse. The left front shows a broken back axis that is severe enough to have caused the coffin bone to tilt backwards. This is called a negative plane coffin bone or a negative palmar angle. With the coffin joint out of alignment, there is excess downward force on the navicular bone, placing it in an unnatural weight bearing position. The dash-line depicts the direction of force down through the limb that passes through the navicular bone. Compare this to the normal alignment in Fig 6.14 where that same line of force is more closely matched with the normal hoof pastern axis.

Fig 6.14 Normal alignment of the hoof pastern axis in the right front, despite the long toe. This illustrates that although a long toe can cause broken back axis, it does not always do so. Broken hoof pastern axis can present complex problems involving ligaments and tendons. When normal trimming and shoeing fails to correct the problem, a more thorough soft tissue assessment by a veterinarian is needed.

this condition. Let's look at some principles of heel pain and place this in the context of what you have learned from previous chapters about optimal hoof care.

Speculative Mechanisms and Risk Factors

There is general agreement that heel pain can be caused by improper loading of the hoof structure. A hoof with poor conformation might cause such loading, or, hoof pain may occur in any foot that is overloaded. Heel pain seems to be frequently associated with off-balance feet, particularly with feet that lack good shock absorbing capacity. Practitioners have observed that predisposing factors for navicular include small feet, under-run heels, or excessively steep, upright heels. All of these conditions can result in excess stress.

There are under-recognized factors that appear to be associated with the onset of navicular. One is the practice of starting a horse in heavy work at two or three years old, before the hoof structures are fully mature. Another is that some horses move too little as they are growing because they are confined to stalls and small paddocks. There are instances where these factors are combined. While these factors have not been studied, practical experience supports the idea that lack of appropriate movement and/or overwork on immature feet predisposes horses to a variety of lameness conditions.

By looking at possible contributing factors, we can speculate about the mechanisms causing pain. For small feet, it may be simply reduced surface area that causes overloading of the hoof. In addition to predisposing a horse to navicular, small feet can also predispose them to laminitis.

At first glance it seems counter intuitive that either low under-run heels or steep upright heels may be associated with navicular, but closer inspection reveals a

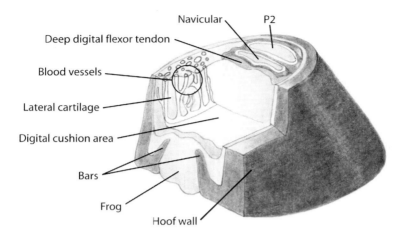

Fig 6.15 This schematic shows one of the key findings in Bowker's navicular research. The lateral cartilage in sound horses is thick with multiple vascular channels running through it. In navicular horses, the lateral cartilage is thin, has few blood vessels, and the existing vessels are all found along the very outer edge rather than distributed throughout the cartilage. Part of Bowker's hypothesis regarding how the foot dissipates energy involves the movement of blood through vessels at the back of the foot.

commonality to these two different imbalances. In each case, shock absorption may be impaired. In under-run feet, the weight bearing points of the heels have migrated forward. The horse lands on heel horn that is below the navicular bone, instead of landing on heels that are further back. The back half of the foot has no bones, and seems designed to play an important role in shock absorption. As discussed in Chapter 3, Dave Duckett's basic balance principle is that hoof function is most efficient with the weight-bearing points of the heels trimmed so they are close to the base of the frog, placing the hoof properly under, rather than in front of, the limb.

In steep upright feet the coffin bone may be tilted forward, which is sometimes a form of phalangeal rotation, as described above in the laminitis section. This overloads the front of the foot and again bypasses the normal shock-absorbing role of hoof structures behind the coffin bone. Upright feet with short pasterns have less range of motion in the fetlock joint than do feet with more sloping hoof pastern axes. Since one of the major mechanisms of shock absorption is joint movement, this upright or "boxy" conformation may predispose to concussion related disorders, navicular being only one possible risk.

Additionally, a steep, tall heel places the frog well above the ground, thus compromising the supportive function of the back half of the foot. The alignment is different than a low under-run heel, but one functional effect may be similar. In both cases the normal loading has been altered.

There are currently no widely available imaging or biopsy techniques available to directly study the inner hoof tissues of live horses. Using feet from cadavers, recent research in Dr. Bowker's laboratory has identified new findings in hooves of navicular feet. One research project compared post-mortem feet of pleasure horses euthanized for

These two photographs illustrate an important concept regarding postural tendency and hoof growth patterns. If you take a group of horses and leave them untrimmed for several months, they may develop different distortions. Some will develop tall heels, some will develop underrun heels. Other horses will develop heels that flare outward, while others will contract inwards. Some toes will dish, others will stay straight. The key to maintaining balance in your horse is to know his tendencies and to prevent them by trimming the part of the hoof that becomes out of place.

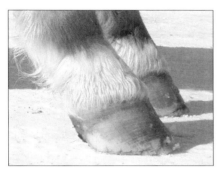

Fig 6.16 This steep hoof of an 8 year old Quarter Horse has a short broken forward pastern that predisposes him to heel pain. This type of foot does not become underrun when it gets long. Nor does it contract. With this much wall height, the frog and sole do not participate in weight bearing, even on soft terrain. With heels this straight and tall, the toe wall laminae are taking more than their share of the load. Additionally, the steep conformation limits the range of motion in the pastern.

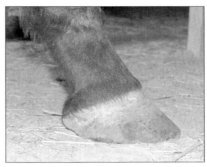

Fig 6.17 This hoof of a 10 year old Thoroughbred has a completely different shape and growth pattern, but also places a horse at risk for heel pain. This hoof has a broken back pastern axis, which places added stress on the navicular area. The heel horn tends to grow forward and become crushed, and the toe quickly becomes too long in between shoeing appointments. Keeping this horse barefoot has allowed for frequent trimming of the toe to maintain improved balance. Even with ideal hoof care, the posture of this horse and the growth tendencies place him at risk of heel pain.

navicular lameness to sound pleasure horses that died for non-hoof related reasons. The previously reported navicular changes were confirmed in this study.

The breakthrough finding in Bowker's project was that navicular feet had additional tissue changes that were not found in the sound feet. The navicular feet had osteoporosis in the arch of the coffin bone, thin lateral cartilages with less blood vessels running through them, and no fibrocartilage in the digital cushion. Each of these differences suggests that the navicular feet had reduced shock absorbing capacity.

Joint movement is one way to absorb shock, which is why you land with a flexed knee when you run. A horse with biomechanically favorable joint angles and good alignment in the hoof pastern axis is able to handle landing forces. In addition to the joint movement, bones perform some shock absorption. The web of lace-like inner bone is able to provide some force attenuation.

If a horse has upright pasterns, he may have compromised shock absorption. If that horse also has thin lateral cartilages and non-resilient digital cushions, he may be further compromised. At this time mechanistic explanations remains purely speculative.

On-going research continues to provide insight into the nature of navicular syndrome and gives the horse community hope that we are beginning to understand the complex nature of navicular disease. We do not have answers to important questions such as: how can we evaluate coffin bone density and the health of the digital cushion and lateral cartilage in live horses? What environmental factors play a role in affected versus sound horses' lives that may account for any of these changes?

Relationship Between Inner and Outer Hoof Structures

Does the appearance of the outer hoof reflect the condition and health of the inner workings of the hoof? Laminitis research suggests that toe wall and white line distortion provide some indication regarding the integrity of the laminar bond. Dave Duckett's studies have shown the relationship between certain external markers and the location of internal structures. Although Robert Bowker's research has found a clear difference in the composition and integrity of inner hoof structures between navicular and non-navicular feet, more research is necessary to understand how this relates to outer hoof form.

This book provides ways to recognize hoof balance and hoof health by a series of external indicators. Healthy feet, as defined by farriers, are balanced with good horn quality and no distortion. Does this mean we should assume that these feet have healthy inner structures? Perhaps it is the good inner structures that explain some of the tough horses – the horses that never go lame no matter how much neglect or abuse they take. Maybe good balance can make up for lack of good inner structure. Or perhaps inner and outer balance are correlated. Studies are underway to investigate these and other unanswered questions.

Prevention and Treatment of Heel Pain

The bottom line for navicular horses is that some aspect of the heel area has either degenerated or was never generated properly in the first place. It is not possible to significantly change upright or low conformation when these postural traits are due to the length and joint conformation of the pastern bones. The horse's feet can only be balanced as well as conformation will allow.

A common factor to all forms of generalized heel pain is that concussion is likely to make the pain more severe and make the underlying condition worse. Whenever a horse alters his way of going to relieve one part of the foot or body from discomfort, eventually the stronger foot is going to be overloaded and will be likely to develop problems. With heel pain, a horse will try to walk on his toes, which in turn can overload the front of the foot and place excessive pressure on the toe wall laminae. Horses initially diagnosed with navicular may eventually develop laminitis.

In this case prevention and treatment have the same goal: to establish good hoof balance. Degeneration as a general expression often suggests an irreversible condition. In reality, there are stages to degeneration just as there are stages to original generation (development). Therefore, if heel pain is identified early enough, it may be reversible. As with any injury, the time needed to heal depends on numerous factors.

Foam Padding for Heel Pain

The application of foam, like with laminitis, can be used to rehabilitate a navicular horse. One key to rehabilitating a navicular horse is to change hoof landing and loading patterns to stop stumbling or toe-stabbing gait. Balanced shoeing may improve soundness in a performance horse that must continue working. Unfortunately, many horses that stay in work become lame again. For a horse given time off, the use of foam padding can offer a more long-lasting solution. The foam padding breaks the cycle of pain, encouraging the horse to load the back of the hoof normally. No studies have been conducted, but there are cases of navicular horses diagnosed as incurable that became sound after treatment with foam padding. Other cases have shown that even without pads, simply rebalancing hooves and keeping them barefoot was enough to allow reversal of navicular symptoms.

While no firm evidence for prevention exists, principles of hoof care presented in this book will provide your horse with the best chances of long term soundness. In addition to well-balanced feet regularly trimmed or shod by a competent farrier, you can take added precautions with a horse known to be at higher risk of navicular.

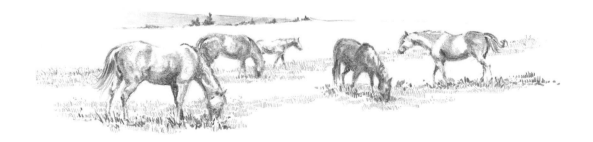

A Holistic Approach

While this chapter has focused on the inner workings of the foot, holistic care is never focused on a single element of wellness. By following the practices laid out in this book, you are already providing holistic care in the prevention of laminitis and navicular. Laminitis and navicular are two afflictions everyone hopes their horse will never face. Drawing on the expertise and support of everyone on your hoof care team will give you the encouragement you need to respond successfully.

Chapter Highlights

- Laminitis is degradation of the laminar junction between the hoof wall and coffin bone. Founder is when the wall and bone move out of alignment.
- There are multiple causes of laminitis: feeding errors, illness, chronic hoof imbalance.
- If not treated immediately, severe laminitis can rapidly become irreversible.
- Laminitis is detectable by clinical signs. X-rays can confirm diagnosis and help guide treatment.
- Laminitis is preventable and curable.
- Navicular syndrome is a chronic condition of heel pain.
- Navicular syndrome is a manageable condition.
- The cause of navicular is unknown. Conformation and hoof imbalance are associated with navicular syndrome.
- Maintaining balanced hoof and horse health will increase the chances of lifelong freedom from navicular or laminitis.

Recommended Reading

Equine Laminitis, Chris Pollitt, BVSc, PhD
Explaining Laminitis and its Prevention, Robert Eustace, BVSc, FRCVS

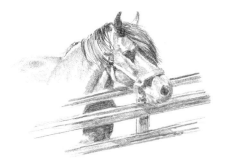

chapter seven

Sound Management

- Hoof Care Team Approach
- Selecting a Farrier
- Trimming and Safety
- Record keeping and Scheduling
- You Are in Control of Your Horse's Health

Sound hoof care management goes a long way toward maintaining a sound horse. Paying attention to the "little" day-to-day things can make all the difference to your horse's comfort and health. This chapter provides a framework on which to build your hoofcare program. Choosing your team, keeping records, having patience, and assuring safety for you and your horse are essential for both the well-being and longevity of the equine-human partnership.

Because the domesticated horse does not encounter the natural forces required to maintain its own feet, as the horse's caretaker you must do the job that nature no longer can. In keeping with the principles of holistic wellness, your hoof care management plan is one aspect of the big picture of equine health. The principles you apply to hoof care will also serve you well in other aspects of horse care. To promote hoof wellness requires vigilance and sound horse husbandry. Initially, many people are daunted by the level of care the domestic hoof requires, and may feel it is too difficult to do alone. By creating your own hoof care team, you will have the support you need.

Support Team

Using the hoof care team approach, you rely on experts to provide specialized assistance and training, and a support network of other people to help you learn about hoof care options and responsibilities. To make the best hoof care choices, you need information. Teamwork will help you to learn the most while providing customized hoof care for your horse. Although the experts will assist you in decision-making, ultimately you, as team leader, are responsible for hoof care decisions.

The support network includes your equine health care practitioners because they will naturally encourage and assist you regarding hoof care decisions. The farrier and veterinarian are core members of the team. Selecting and keeping a good farrier is emphasized in this chapter, though the same principles should be applied to searching for and communicating with other equine professionals. Additional team members include any or all of the following: chiropractor, dentist, physical therapist, acupressurist, massage therapist, and nutritionist.

For many, the most significant support network will come from other horse people like yourself who have been through the experience of taking charge of their own horse's hoof health.

There are growing communities of horse people who are helping each other in this uncharted realm of hoof care responsibility. If you find yourself facing the unnerving decision of respectfully opting out of orthodox hoof care, you will be able to find support and guidance from others who have been there before you.

Selecting a Farrier

For most horse people, doing their own hoof care is neither practical nor desirable, so hiring a professional is the normal course of action. Even those who do some of their own hoof care need a professional occasionally. Selecting the right professional for your horse's needs is not easy. You have probably read articles in popular horse publications on selecting a farrier. They are full of sensible advice: find someone trained, qualified, professional, well-mannered and so on. These are laudable traits, but may not be sufficient credentials to meet your horse's needs.

You do not need to know all that the experts know in order to evaluate them. What you need to know is how to distinguish a genuinely knowledgeable, capable person from one who may be under-qualified to work on your horse.

Is your farrier willing to acknowledge your interest in the process of your horse's hoof care? Does your farrier make the effort to keep you informed about your horse's feet? Try not to bombard your farrier with questions about new trim methods or a controversial hoof care protocol you have recently heard about. Farriers are usually on a busy schedule. Develop a relationship with your farrier. Once you have communicated your level of understanding about the hoof and your farrier knows that you have put some thought and study into it, you are more likely to have fruitful conversation.

Farriers should be able to describe their approach to hoof care. If their description includes balance, that's a plus, but without further qualification this statement means little – every farrier has their own understanding of balance. You need to inquire further and find out what schools of thought and training methods influence their work. Be wary of claims that all feet should be at a certain angle, have a certain look to the hairline, have frogs on the ground, or be so many inches long. One-size-fits-all theories might lead to dangerous mistakes.

If your veterinarian diagnoses your horse with a particular lameness, ask your farrier about advantages and disadvantages of the different options for treating this condition. If the farrier responds with vague or evasive answers: "This works because I've seen it work before" or "I've been doing this for 30 years and have won lots of awards"– this may not be the person with whom you want to work. Listen for broad generalizations or "trademark" technique, such as making all toes square or using the same shape and type of shoe on every horse. These may be red flags.

Many professionals keep up with new research and clinical evidence by attending continuing education clinics or reading professional journals, and can respond to your questions with knowledge. Ask specific questions. Find out what they know, not just what they think. If a farrier dismisses particular methods out-of-hand, or is unwilling to discuss a full range of options, you may want to continue your search.

Having successfully completed a formal training program may be a good criterion for selecting a farrier. Yet plenty of excellent farriers learned the trade from apprenticeship, never attending a school or becoming certified. Farriers graduating from the same shoeing school may not be like-minded or have the same caliber of professionalism. Having many years of experience is good, although there are farriers with decades on the job who have never learned how to balance a foot. You need to know something about the quality and level of that experience and how it has shaped the approach that particular farrier takes in his work. Finding an experienced certified farrier is not the end-point of your selection process, it is only a place to start.

Certification does not necessarily guarantee that a hoofcare professional is qualified. However, American Farrier Association certification means that the farrier has been tested to a nationally recognized standard. In the case of trimmer certifications, there are widely varying and sometimes conflicting standards with no national accreditation. Therefore, you must be equally careful and discerning in choosing either farrier or trimmer. Look beyond the badge. In the end, you have to be confident that your farrier is doing the right thing for your horse, and comfortable asking them to do just that.

How to Keep a Farrier

You have the right to interview and choose the best farrier for your horse. In their own way, farriers also interview and choose their clients. Long-time farrier Henry Heymering, president of the Guild of Professional Farriers noted the following attributes possessed by good clients.

Good clients have well trained horses. Unruly horses are dangerous to themselves, to the farrier, and to you. Some farriers are willing to work on such horses, but will charge you more. Other farriers will not work on

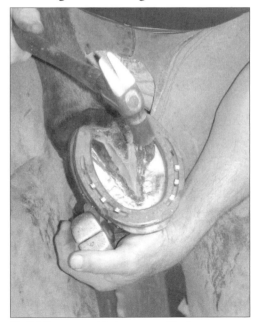

Fig 7.1 Do your part to keep a good farrier.

> **One-size-fits-all theories might lead to dangerous mistakes.**

uncooperative horses. There are horses that are cooperative with a certain farrier but not with another. Look for a good personality match between farrier and horse. If you have a horse that needs a slower, gentler approach to nailing or hoof holding position, find someone willing to adjust to your horse.

Designate an area of your barn for safe farrier work. Clean, open, quiet, well lit, with a level hard surface – concrete or hard rubber mats are best. If you have the luxury of designing your own barn, be sure to include a good "hoof care station".

Be ready when the farrier arrives. The horse should be caught, tied, brushed, and clean when the farrier arrives. This ought to go without saying, but it is a common oversight.

Make and keep regular appointments. You cannot expect a busy farrier to come to your barn on a moments notice. For an emergency, such as a lost shoe right before a competition, most farriers will make a special effort for a good client. In general, principles of hoof care rest upon preventive measures. Regularly scheduled appointments at the interval you and your farrier deem ideal for your horse contribute greatly to your horse's long-term soundness.

Doing Your Own Trimming

You may want to learn how to rasp sound feet and maintain balance. Some farriers are happy to teach you trim basics. There are farriers who specialize in conducting clinics to teach basic trimming.

> **Using a knife or nippers properly requires considerable experience and should be done only by a farrier.**

Using a knife or nippers properly requires considerable experience and should be done only by a farrier. Re-establishing balance, particularly in a diseased foot, is complicated and should be done only by a farrier as well. If your horse has sound, balanced bare feet, you can maintain them just by rasping. With proper training from a qualified hoofcare professional, this is a safe and effective way to maintain hoof balance between farrier visits.

Safety

Your farrier probably makes it look easy, but working on a horse's feet is physically demanding and can be hazardous – there are basic guidelines you must follow. It may be tempting to stick tools in your pockets or use a tool belt to keep everything handy, but it's not a good idea. There is a reason why farriers keep everything off their body except the knives, which are secured in thick leather protected pockets. If you get knocked

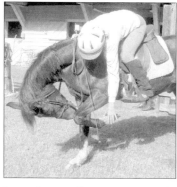

down with a tool in your pocket, the tool could injure you or your horse. As you know from watching farriers work, it is a challenge to keep tools both close at hand and in a safe position.

Hoof care is physically hard. You may be tempted to sit on a chair or stool while trimming, but it is poor practice, as the chances of being hurt are greatly increased. You can buy stands with cradles for holding the hoof. These offer a relatively safe alternative to the traditional farrier stance provided you have a well-trained horse. The horse's comfort is essential. A comfortable horse is safer. Do not put yourself or your horse at risk in the interests of your own comfort. If you cannot find a way to stand up and trim your horse's feet, you need to hire a professional.

Record Keeping

Detailed notes on your horse's normal way of going, and the bumps, bruises and other signs of stress that come and go will help you recognize deviations more readily. For example, when your horse is in training, early signs of metabolic or musculoskeletal stress will tell you to rest your horse for a few days. If you are not accustomed to looking closely and do not establish a normal baseline for your horse, you could easily miss early signs.

An isolated observation may seem meaningless when you first notice it. Write it down nonetheless. Patterns emerge when you keep good records. If you notice a bump on your horse one day, or a slight limp, or a day when he does not have much of an appetite, write it down.

Good records will provide you with an answer to one of the most common questions a veterinarian or farrier asks: "How long has this been like this?" If you inspect your horse closely on a routine basis, you can determine when new symptoms appear. It is so common for a horse to have "mild" symptoms such as slight limping, leg swelling, etc. that most people do not track them. If the horse ever needs veterinary attention, these previously mild insults might be important history for you to relate to the practitioner.

What information should you record? Keep veterinary and farrier records of your own. Veterinarians keep records on all clients, as do quite a few farriers. It helps to have your own copies of this information. Keep the records in the barn, clearly labeled and accessible to anyone looking after your horse.

The rate of your horse's hoof growth can be tracked. With frequent hoof care appointments, you may notice that feet not only grow faster but also wear more slowly since healthy, good quality horn is tough. Some wear does take place, thus the amount of hoof removed at each appointment is not necessarily the full amount that has grown since the previous trimming.

One way to gauge exactly how much horn growth has occurred each month is to make a mark on the hoof wall and measure its downward progress over time. Make a small notch exactly one inch below the hairline in the center of the dorsal hoof wall. Record the date, and then simply measure its distance from the hairline a month later. Do this over a period of months, making a new notch as necessary when the old one reaches the ground surface. As you track this over a year, you may find variations in growth rate. By keeping track of your horses shoeing, feeding, work, and medical history you may find significant correlations.

Paying close attention to the feet will lead you to pay close attention to the rest of the horse. The following are commonly found across the domestic horse population: hoof-dragging, slight wall or sole bruising, difficultly holding the feet up for the farrier, stretched white lines. These signs are so frequently seen that many experienced horsemen believe they are insignificant. As discussed previously, these signs offer clues to early hoof and other health problems.

If you or your farrier notice an imbalance developing in a horse that had previously been staying well balanced, check your records to see if you have notes about any movement problems. An equine chiropractic exam might find the cause quickly, and the feet can be returned to normal balance.

> **…commonly found across the domestic horse population: hoof-dragging, slight wall or sole bruising, difficultly holding the feet up for the farrier, stretched white lines. These signs are so frequently seen that many experienced horsemen believe they are insignificant…these signs offer clues to early hoof and other health problems.**

Scheduling

Each horse is an individual and scheduling hoof care will be influenced by a horse's particular needs. The reality of the farrier industry is that in order to schedule efficiently for business purposes, farriers normally pick a particular interval that works well for the average horse. Sometimes the needs are shaped by the rider, trainer, or farrier scheduling preferences rather than by consideration of the horse's hoof health. The industry recommends hoofcare on a five to eight week schedule. This would seem to be a good compromise for everyone. Within this five to eight week schedule, farriers can have a large client base, people are used to paying for hoof care on this schedule, and horses appear to do well with this arrangement.

Your horse may not be the average horse. Many horses do better if attended to more frequently. Horses that do acceptable work when shod every other month may do even better if shod more frequently.

Farriers who keep horses on tighter schedules have observed that hoof may grow faster if trimmed or reshod more often. Only tiny amounts need to be rasped, this stimulates the feet enough to cause more growth than when left untouched. Growth rate often varies with the season or the amount of work the horse is doing. However, chronically slow growth may indicate ill health.

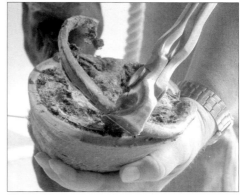

Fig 7.2 When this much horn is removed in one appointment, your horse may benefit from more frequent farrier visits.

You know that tracking hoof growth can reveal important clues about hoof and overall horse health. The other essential reason for keeping growth rate records is to customize your hoof care scheduling. Healthy hooves average one-quarter to one-half an inch of growth per month. If your horse grows one-quarter of an inch in a month, he may do very well being reshod every six weeks. If he grows one-half inch per month, a four-week schedule would be better. And, if barefoot, the rate of wear will depend on exposure to abrasive surfaces.

The goal of frequent trimming is to maintain consistent balance rather than significantly change the hoof length at each appointment

The goal of frequent trimming is to maintain consistent balance rather than significantly change the hoof length at each appointment. Hoof length is an integral part of balance. If your farrier only has to remove a small amount of horn to balance the hoof, then you know the hoof was fairly well balanced before the trim.

Your Horse's Health is in Your Hands

People have horses for different reasons and hoof care practitioners must acknowledge this fact. When the horse's job is high performance and there is no time for lengthy rehabilitation, then the obligation of the farrier is to present trimming and shoeing options that will minimize pain and maximize performance immediately. When the horse is not required to work right away then the farrier can present a full range of rehabilitation options.

Do not allow yourself to be pressured into treatment plans that seem inappropriate for you and your horse's needs. When you hire a hoof care practitioner who prefers to keep horses barefoot, you may be made to feel bad for wanting shoes. Only *you* can truly determine what your horse needs. If you know your horse needs to go down the road to stay happy, all the alleged healing that can come from being barefoot is irrelevant if your horse can't work without shoes.

At first, it might be intimidating to be the leader of your horse's hoof care team. Know that you have the support of professional equine healthcare providers. You also have a valuable resource in the social network surrounding horse care. Turn to your friends who are grappling with similar issues regarding the best methods of solving problems. After you have gathered information from your support team and reviewed all your records, trust yourself and have the courage to do whatever is needed to keep your horse sound. Your full participation in meeting your horse's hoof care needs is essential for whole horse wellness. You are the spokesperson for your horse. Do not let him down.

Chapter highlights

- Hooves require frequent attention to make up for the absence of natural conditions.
- You are responsible for providing the horse with hoof care that mimics, to some extent, what has been taken away by domestication.
- Good horsemanship requires basic knowledge of the hoof.
- Record keeping is essential.
- A key to ideal hoof health is frequency of farrier appointments.

Recommended Reading

The Equine Foot, Fran Jurga
The Natural Hoof, Jaime Jackson

chapter eight

Action Gallery

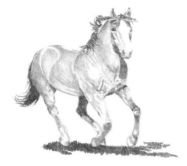

Everyone is familiar with shod horses doing well in all sports since the majority of sport horses are shod. You hear little about the performance horses who are doing the same things well or better barefoot. It's not that they aren't out there – they are, but have not reached the public eye as yet.

This chapter is about barefoot performers. While the shod vs barefoot debate will rage indefinitely, there is little doubt that more horses could be sound and barefoot than currently are. If you have read everything up to this point, you know that science and research do not dispute this, even if they aren't ready to support it. This chapter is not designed to provide scientific evidence, it is meant to provide hope and inspiration for everyone who is wondering, "what if…"

These are stories of people and horses who were willing to buck conventional wisdom by going barefoot in the face of everyone who said "it couldn't be done."

The road to going barefoot varies for each of these cases. No conclusions can be derived from these stories but they may help convince horse owners that it is worth a try. These are stories from people just like you, with horses just like yours.

There are a growing number of barefoot trimmers trained and certified according to different views of how the hoof works. Choosing to go barefoot is not without risk, as it's easy to mistake passionate belief for authoritative knowledge, especially if you are desperate to help a lame horse. Whether farrier or trimmer, you must choose your hoofcare professional with the same care you would choose a surgeon.

Whatever the situation for each horse, the common thread in all of these cases is high owner participation, improved performance for the horse, and enhanced horse-human relationships.

We do not know how much our horses are capable of doing until we give them a chance to show us.

A Tribute

To understand developments in barefoot hoof care and the directions it may take, look to the pioneering work of Jaime Jackson, founder of the American Association of Natural Hoof Care Practitioners. Jackson has spent the past two decades blazing a trail into the future with his barefoot hoof care guidelines based on the wild horse model.

Jaime Jackson, a man ahead of his time, is an active participant in shaping today's hoof care landscape. Jackson did what no one else had done before or since

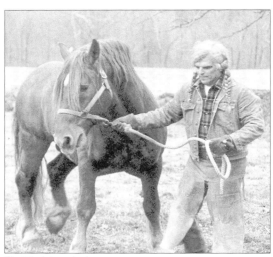

Fig 8.1 Jaime Jackson

his work in the 1980s. He conducted field work among wild horses, living as a true animal anthropologist amongst his study subjects. Jackson painstakingly observed and documented what he saw, much of which had never before been reported. This is a special tribute to Jaime Jackson and his contribution to hoof care. Thank you Jaime, for your work. You coined the term "Power Trim." What you learned from the wild horses, and what you have shared with the rest of us, is indeed powerful.

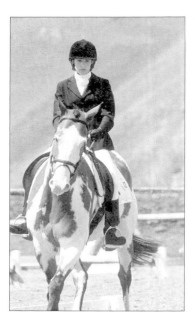

Fig 8.2 Willy and Gisele

Willy, Dressage Master

Willy, a 14 year old registered American Paint Horse, suffered a suspensory injury in 2000, and subsequently had a series of mysterious lamenesses. He was diagnosed a year later with mild navicular syndrome. Today, Willy is barefoot, sound, and back competing in upper level dressage shows. Willy has the same farrier now as when he was shod. Gisele Olson, Willy's owner summarizes her experience.

> Willy was boarded at a premier equestrian facility and lived what I thought was the "high life." He spent his nights in a roomy box stall, his days in a paddock. He ate the newest scientific feeds twice a day; my family spent a lot of money for his trainer, his farrier, and his veterinarian. Willy and I competed in dressage shows around the

region and were preparing for regional championships when he was injured. The next year became an odyssey of searching for answers to his perplexing and persistent lameness. With nothing else to lose, I tried the heretical: I directed his farrier to take off his horseshoes and turned him out full time in a pasture with a small herd of other horses. Willy's miraculous recovery the following year forced me to rethink everything I had been taught about caring for a performance horse. I encourage all horse owners to learn about natural horse care and to do whatever they can to apply the principles to their horses. It is the least we can do for an animal that, for some amazing reason, has agreed to let us be part of its life.

Royal Code, High Performance at the Top of His Sport

Royal Code is a 10 year old Thoroughbred gelding who has been barefoot since 2002 competing at preliminary level eventing. The fences are big and the courses are technically difficult. The horse must be able to perform well on variable footing in dressage, cross-country, and stadium jumping. Kendall DeRoo shares her story.

Since our horses have been barefoot, their traction has been exceptional. Stumbling, while never a major problem for any of them, has virtually disappeared. A barefoot horse has more control because he can feel what's happening.

At an event where stadium jumping was held in a grass field after a day of heavy rain, Royal, jumping barefoot, was one of only two horses out of 20 to jump clean.

The intense environment of competition highlighted all the improvements I saw in the horse at home. He galloped and jumped in all kinds of footing. He improved in posture and carriage, which improved his dressage ability and presentation. His recovery was exceptional.

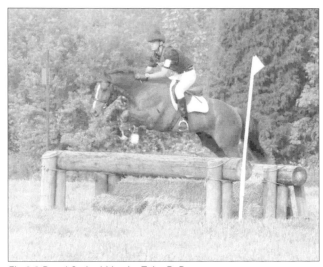

Fig 8.3 Royal Code ridden by Tyler DeRoo

From Mounted Patrol To Winter Sleigh Driving

Gunner is an 11 year old Quarter Horse gelding, a retired cutting horse, he is now used for police work on the streets of Jackson Hole, Wyoming. In the winter, he remains barefoot while pulling a sleigh. Gunner's owner, Jamie Cline, has found his way of going to be smoother and safer when working the streets in bare feet.

After removing my horse's shoes and riding barefoot, I noticed a significant difference in his stride. He moves so much more comfortably. Since I use him to patrol downtown with a "citizen's mounted unit" he has much better traction on the streets with bare feet. I have no fear that his feet will slip out from underneath him, which happened when he was shod.

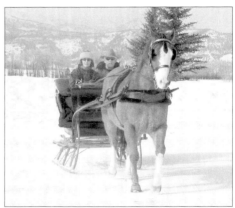

Fig 8.4 Jamie and Gunner

Barrel Racing, Big O Style

Melissa Rider has a long background as a barrel racer. She is successfully competing her barefoot quarter horses Black Jack and Big O in this demanding sport. Melissa competes in the American West 4D circuit.

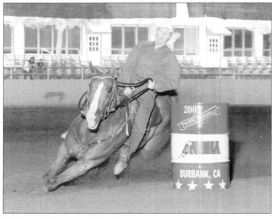

I have barrel raced for many years, and there is no comparison between the feel of a barefoot horse and the feel of a shod horse. A barefoot horse does not slide on hard ground. Since going barefoot, I have not had a barrel horse so much as slip while turning. It is my opinion that if you have two barrel horses of equal physical ability, the barefoot horse will out-run and out-maneuver the shod horse.

Fig 8.5 Melissa and Big O

Xena, Queen of Cutting

Xena is a 7 year old Quarter Horse mare who performs barefoot. Her owner Jamie Cline was previously cutting on shod horses and has noticed an improvement while riding a barefoot horse.

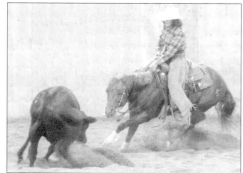

Her performance and soundness have been enhanced going without shoes. She can stop and turn with increased traction. Many cutters complain about a hard packed ope up area. I never have to worry about that since my horse does not have the added concussion that steel shoes cause.

Fig 8.6 Jamie and Xena

The Long Distance Horse

Growing numbers of long distance riders have found that barefoot horses do as well, or better, during competition. Just as importantly, these horses do distinctly better after the competition than they did when they wore shoes. Whether they are going 25 or 100 miles in a day, whether they go at a leisurely pace or fast enough to finish in the top 10, long distance riders are finding out that the barefoot horse is capable of an impressive performance.

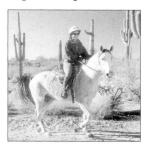

Fig 8.7 Just Spin to Win, wearing Swiss Horse Boots on the front feet. Ridden by Sara Goodnick.

Endurance Racing – Limited Distance

Just Spin to Win is a 6 year old Arab mare, owned by Kirt Lander, a Natural Hoof Care Practitioner who trained with Jaime Jackson at the American Association of Natural Hoofcare Practitioners. His horses routinely finish top 10 in 25, 30 and 50-mile endurance races. Kirt believes that barefoot performance horses benefit in body and hoof, and outperform shod horses.

I think that the heart rate of barefoot endurance horses comes down a bit quicker than the shod horse. I have proven to myself that with the right hoof care and living conditions, there is nothing to be lost in terms of performance and only benefits to be gained in terms of health, soundness, safety and longevity. I think the barefoot competitior horse is actually going to be raising the bar.

Zahara is an endurance horse living in Florida where she gladly races barefoot. Zahara's owner Maria Villenevue had not heard of "the barefoot movement" or read any books about it. She had one simple reason for trying the mare barefoot. Zahara was interfering, and no matter what the farrier did, the horse always interfered during races. So the farrier removed the shoes and kept the same trim. Zahara stopped interfering, and has been doing well ever since. She is a regular top 10 finisher in 50 mile endurance races.

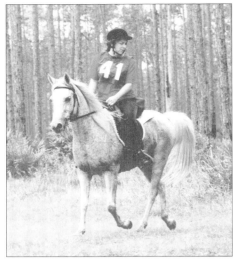
Fig 8.8 Zahara and Maria

Endurance Racing – Long Distance

United States Equestrian Team endurance rider and long-time competitive distance rider Darolyn Butler-Dial has taken barefoot competition horses to the top of this challenging sport. Her top horses occasionally wear shoes or boots for a few of the one-day hundreds on the most demanding terrain. Darolyn's endurance horses routinely finish in the top 10, often winning with the fastest time and/or the Best Condition score. She is in the top 10 for lifetime miles ridden and will have completed 25,000 miles of competition riding in 2005. Darolyn describes the changes she has seen since going barefoot.

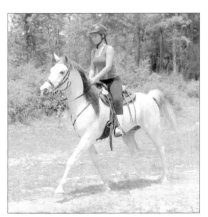
Fig 8.9 One of Darolyn's endurance horses DJB Cytron ridden by Meghan Dunn.

Since we started racing horses barefoot, we have noticed they maintain healthy legs, no windpuffs, and are not as likely to have suspensory or other tendon problems. The horses have no interfering or forging. We see improved heart rate recoveries at the vet checks and sound feet after the races, meaning no distorted hoof ring growth showing up a month later. There is almost no stocking up the day after a competition or after long hauls in the trailer.

Pleasure Riding and Companion Horse – A Rocky Road But Finally Barefoot Sound

Skeeter, an 8 year old Quarter Horse, has had a long and painful journey. In 2000 he was head-bobbing lame at the walk, diagnosed with severe navicular syndrome. His owner Barb Hoskinson tried several different hoof care options. The horse was kept well-shod by a competent farrier for several months but was still lame. An inappropriate barefoot trim caused a setback, but Barb decided to try barefoot again with a different farrier. After 2 years of slow improvement, Skeeter has remained free of hoof boots and support pads for over a year. Barb has been through a lot with this horse, and has the following to share with other owners who might be in a similar situation.

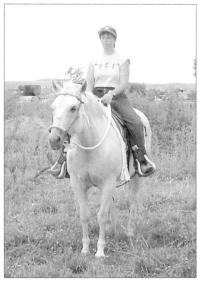

Fig 8.10 Skeeter and Barb

> There is a time for shoes but that should not be the norm. From what I have observed, horses can do better without shoes. Horses give us their all, no questions asked. They go until they can't go anymore. We owe them the same if something goes wrong, we need to explore every single avenue to get them back to where they were. It may take a long time and we need to stick with them through thick and thin. This means we, as their caretakers, need to look outside the box and not be afraid to go by our gut feelings and what we think the horse is telling us.

Halter Horses Don't Need Shoes

Jean Munninghoff shows several top level Quarter Horses with out shoes. They do well and she comments on her experience:

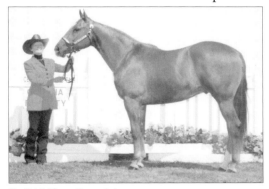

Fig 8.11 Macmito and Jean

> No one at the shows realize my horses are barefoot unless I point it out, and they are amazed. I am the only one, as far as I know, who shows a barefoot horse, with the exception of weanlings and most yearlings, in AQHA.

Carriage Driving and Combined Driving From Minis To Morgans

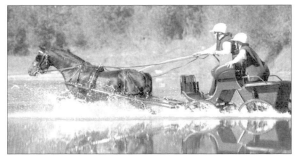
Fig 8.12 Lad and Deb

Lad is a 12 year old all-around athlete, competing barefoot in multiple sports, the most physically demanding of which is combined driving. He competes at Preliminary level in Combined Driving Events, having no trouble with the 15 km Marathon part of the event that takes the horses over roads and tracks with variable terrain, including rocks and gravel.

Lad's owner Deb Harper has fun with her barefoot stallion as well as her flashy miniature gelding, River.

> I have found that you need to condition on the terrain you are going to encounter. I ride Lad on our gravel dykes, haul in gravel to his paddock by his gateways, and drive him on the gravel shoulders of our roads whenever I condition on the streets.
>
> Riverdance is my miniature gelding. River competes at training level in combined driving events where they offer a special division for Very Small Equines. River has been the Hi Score Dressage horse a couple of times (against horses of all sizes) and has also won an Indoor Trial (beat out a 16 hand Welsh Cob stallion, a Friesien and other large horses). Lad and River are often the Best Dressage or Reserve Best- its like this big brother-little brother rivalry.

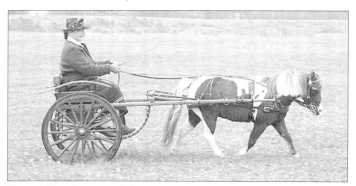
Fig 8.13 Riverdance and Deb

These are just a few chronicles of horses doing what they do best, and doing it barefoot. They are meant to inspire you, to show you that there are fewer boundaries to having your horse perform than you may have believed. For every story here, there are hundreds more waiting to be told.

More performers

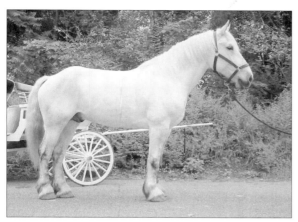

Fig 8.14 This professional carriage horse, Milo, works on pavement. His tough feet have great traction and never get chipped, flared, flat or sore, problems that often plague heavy horses working on hard roads.

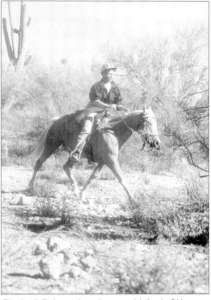

Fig 8.15 Paloma is a 6 year old Arab-QH mare ridden by Donna Blanchette. The mare had been barefoot for one year before this race. Her owner says she will "stomp over just about anything and does not need hoof boots even for rocky terrain."

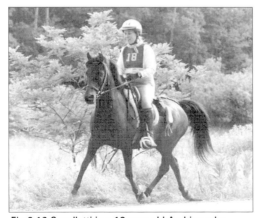

Fig 8.16 Cavalletti is a 10-year old Arabian who competes barefoot in 3-day hundred-mile races. She won the 3-Florida 100 mile competitive ride barefoot. She is an endurance horse and wears shoes for the one-day hundreds. Her owner, Sue Greenall is a top US Endurance Team rider who finds that alternating between barefoot and shoeing meets the needs of her horses.

109

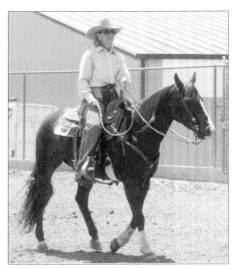

Fig 8.17 Little Bit is a reining horse. She is an 8-year old QH mare whose owner Phebe Peterson decided to try a novel set-up. The horse wears typical reining horse shoes on the hind feet – called sliders, these are special low traction steel shoes that help the horse perform a slide. On the front feet this mare is barefoot. Bare feet in front seem to help her stabilize her front end, allowing the hind feet to work even better in the slide.

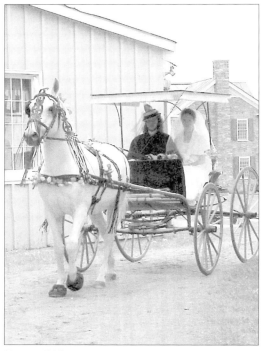

Fig 8.18 Eddie is a 27 year old Arab gelding, used for pleasure riding and driving. He can be barefoot on soft footing and wears Old Mac boots to be comfortable on gravel roads.

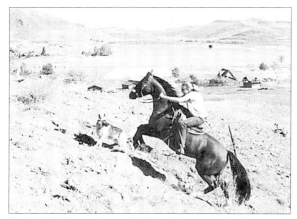

Fig 8.19 Bud is a 10 year old QH gelding owned by Colorado farrier Sheila McAttee. Bud is sound and strong on the tough Colorado terrain, happy to canter or trot over rocky, trappy footing without any trouble or discomfort.

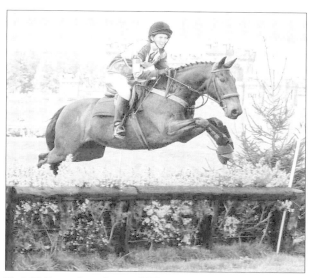

Fig 8.20 Barney is an 8 year old Thoroughbred cross gelding that events barefoot. His owner Deane Roberts lives in Scotland, where she and Barney have qualified for the National Horse Trials Championships.

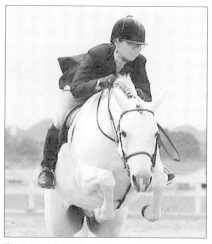

Fig 8.21 Jubilee is a 13 year old Welsh Pony who has never had shoes on in his life. He competes hunter over fences, western pleasure and trail classes as well as English pleasure and halter classes at breed shows. He shows extensively on the "A" circuit.

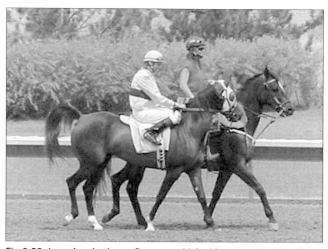

Fig 8.22 Justa Inspiration, a five-year-old Arabian mare, is a barefoot racehorse.

Should your horse be barefoot? Well, that's a decision for you, your horse, and your team. But remember the stories from this chapter when somebody tells you that a horse can't do "that" without shoes. You can be pretty sure that whatever sport or equine activity you can think of, somewhere out there, a horse is already doing it barefoot.

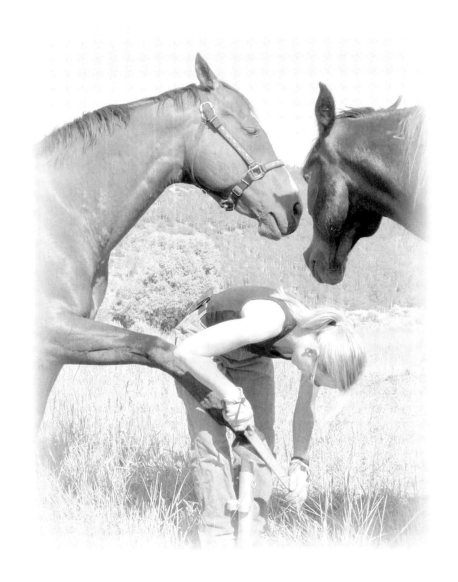

Summary

This book has shared with you multiple ways to evaluate hoof health and approach hoof care. With the diversity of occupations our horses have today, there is no single method of care or equine lifestyle that is right for all. However, a common goal shared by horsemen and horse health practitioners is soundness. In order to achieve and maintain soundness, the first step in hoof care is to balance the foot. Whether shod or barefoot, an off-balance horse will biomechanically and metabolically perform at less than full capacity.

Rather than endorsing any single method for achieving soundness, this book has presented principles to help you assess and choose from a variety of trimming and shoeing methods, and has given you new tools for understanding your horse's feet and taking charge of hoof care.

Holistic hoof care is about building soundness rather than treating a specific lameness. Strict trim guidelines, shoeing beliefs, or particular living arrangements for horses do not define holistic hoof care. Techniques are an important part of holistic care, but there are no "holistic techniques". Rather, holistic hoof care depends on the approach and goals of hoof care that include treating the causes of illness rather than treating only symptoms.

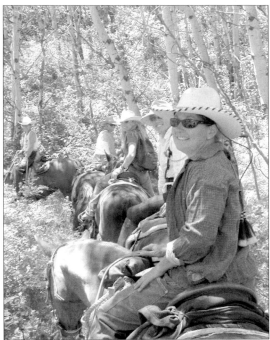

Treatment of lameness may or may not involve special trimming or special shoeing. It is a common misunderstanding to think that holistic hoof care means no shoes will ever be used, just as it is a common misunderstanding to think that a holistic veterinarian will never use drugs or surgery. As caretaker of your horse, your job is to find experts who can help you identify the horse's needs. To that end, you want to find equine practitioners whose approach to health and healing commands your respect. As the needs of the horse and owner change, the holistic farrier will continually adjust the hoofcare technique to match.

The information in this book has shown you why a customized approach

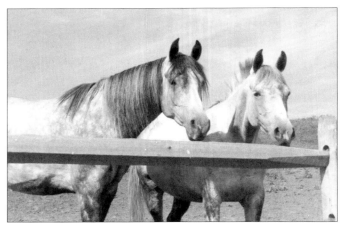

to hoof care is important. Any given method for trimming or shoeing can have radically diverse effects on different horses. Two horses with similar looking feet could each require a different type of trim due to their individual circumstances.

Knowing some anatomy, and armed with your 11-point checklist for hoof assessment, you possess the knowledge and appropriate language to discuss your horse's hoof health with your professional equine practitioners. You are familiar with key concepts in hoof care, such as Duckett's balance principles, which have given you a frame of reference for understanding many of the "new" theories out there today.

You know about recent research on laminitis and navicular. You are prepared to critically assess claims about hoof balance, whether you read them online or in research journals.

The foundation of maintaining hoof health is that your horse gets frequent and consistent hoof care, whether shod or barefoot. This will insure that you are maintaining or evolving, rather than radically changing, your horse's balance. Balanced hooves, balance in feeding, a balanced lifestyle and a strong relationship between you, your horse and your team are the keys to soundness.

Perpetual balance is a possibility for all horses. Understanding that hoof care is an essential part of good horsemanship, you are now ready and able to provide a higher level of hoof care service for your horse. Equipped with the knowledge gained from reading this book, you owe it to your horse to continue building your understanding of horse health from the ground up.

The form on the following page is for you to use with your horses (photocopy it onto card stock). It is designed for recording detailed information about a single foot (identify which foot by circling the labeled outline at the top right of the page). You may choose to fill out information on all four feet initially and then use one page for the whole horse if there is minimal information to record. To help you remember what to look for, the form contains a list of key words taken from the checklist in Chapter 3.

HOOF REPORT CARD

Horse: _____

Date: _____

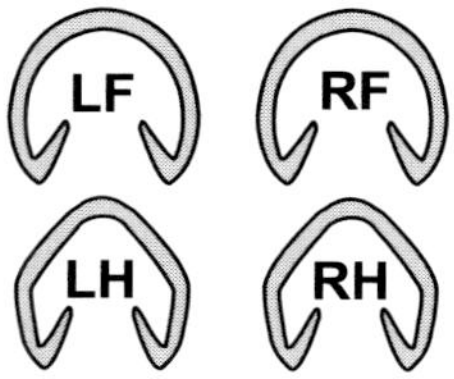

LF RF
LH RH

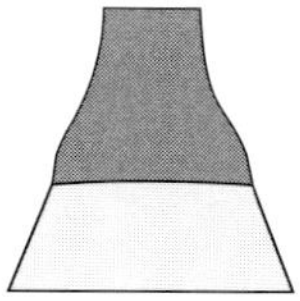

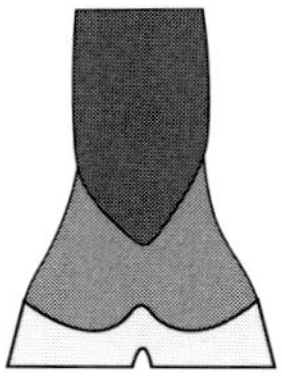

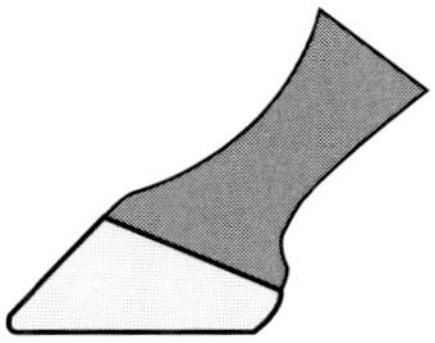

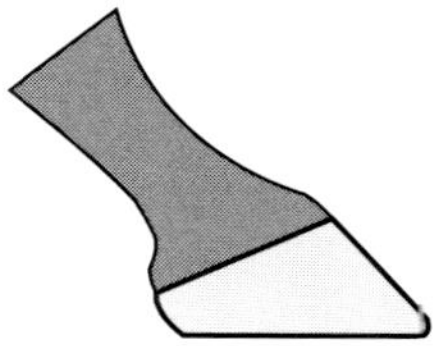

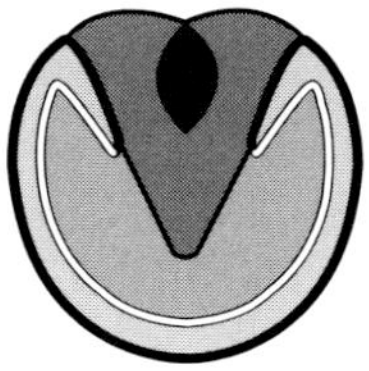

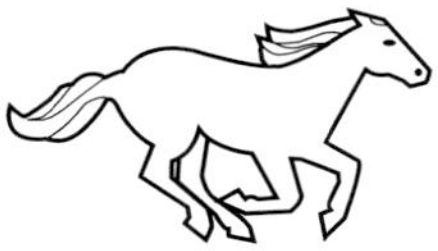

Stance/way of going

Hoof/pastern axis

Hairline

Toe/heel length & angle

Hoof shape

Balance:
 -solar proportions
 -mediolateral
 -symmetry

Frog

Sole

Bar

White line

Hoof/shoe wear pattern

©2004 Lancaster Equine

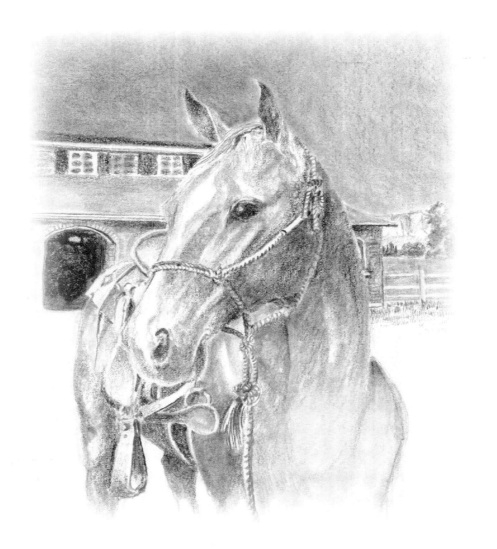

Selected Resources

There is a wealth of resources available on the internet. Below is a listing of a few of the websites created by the current leaders in hoof care. These sites will open up a practically endless exploration of links, web rings, chat rooms, and support groups for any hoof care issue you can imagine. While these websites contain a wealth of information, "consumer beware" should be a guiding principle.

As in any profession, there are plenty of people dispensing advice, and some of them are "arm-chair farriers" – people who have never trimmed or shod a foot, may not have seen very many feet, but are certain about how it should be done. You now have the tools to evaluate their claims and assess the appropriateness of any trimming or shoeing practice for your horse.

www.hoofcare.com Website of Hoofcare and Lameness: Journal of Equine Foot Science. Provides information regarding the world of horse feet. Includes links to other sites. Archives of articles. Books and videos for sale.

www.hopeforsoundness.com Complete information center for Natural Balance Trimming and Shoeing. Many products available, including First Alert Kit and Instructional Video for laminitis emergency treatment. Padding for laminitic horses, designed by Gene Ovnicek, is available on his Natural Balance website. Similar products have been designed by others. To date many horse owners have found that other products are expensive and/or not widely available. Owners have found the solution to customizing their own hoof pads using materials from home building supply or camping stores. You can buy inexpensive insulation foam and follow Natural Balance guidelines for applying it. You can find flooring foam or packaging material that can be made into hoof pads. Owner support groups on the internet are full of creative tips for making hoof pads or boots out of inexpensive easily obtainable material.

www.aanhcp.org American Association of Natural Hoof Care Practitioners. Organization founded by pioneer of natural hoof and horse care, Jaime Jackson.

www.star-ridge.com Owner resources, hoof boots, and tools for trimming can be found at Jaime Jackson's site as well as other barefoot hoof care sites.

www.tribeequus.com Natural hoof care information and links to a webring.

www.thehorseshoof.com Newsletter and informational website about barefoot hoof care and trimming.

www.horsescience.com Freeze dried hoof anatomy models for sale, plus teaching and learning aids.

www.hoofjack.com Recommended popular hoof stand.

www.horseholdup.com A hoof cradle especially helpful for holding up hind legs.

www.lancasterequine.com Includes Hoof Care Record forms available for download, an expanded bibliography on hoof research, and more hoof care information.

www.tallgrasspublishers.com or www.animalacupressure.com Holistic animal healthcare training programs and learning tools including: books, meridian charts, and videos. Offers links to other holistic animal healthcare sites. See this site to order additional copies of *The Sound Hoof: Horse Health from the Ground Up*.

Selected References

Chapter 2

Bowker, Robert M. 2003. The Growth and Adaptive Capabilities of the Hoof Wall and Sole: Functional Changes in Response to Stress. In *Proceedings of the 49th Annual Convention of the American Association of Equine Practitioners*, 49:146-168. New Orleans: AAEP.

Bowker, Robert. 1996. Sensation in the Equine Foot. *Hoofcare and Lameness Journal of Equine Foot Science*, no. 67.

Hallab, N.J., H.A. Hogan, and D.M. Hood. 1991. Determining the Mechanical Properties of Equine Laminar Corium Tissue. *The Equine Athlete* 4, no. 4: 13-18.

Hood, David M., Danny Taylor, and Ilka Wagner. 2001. Effects of ground surface deformability, trimming, and shoeing on quasistatic hoof loading patterns in horses. *American Journal of Veterinary Research* 62, no. 6: 895-900.

Ovnicek, Gene, John B. Erfle, and Duncan F. Peters. 1995. Wild Horse Hoof Patterns Offer a Formula for Preventing and Treating Lameness. *Annual Convention Proceedings of the American Association of Equine Practitioners* 41: 258-260.

Chapter 3

Duckett, Dave. 1988. External Reference Points of the Equine Hoof. *Original Manuscript*

Ovnicek, Gene. 2003. Natural Balance Trimming and Shoeing. In *Diagnosis and Management of Lameness in the Horse*, ed. Mike W. Ross and Sue J. Dyson:271-273. New York: Saunders.

Chapter 4

Colles, C.M. 1989. The relationship of frog pressure to heel expansion. *Equine Veterinary Journal* 21, no. 1: 13-16.

Dyhre-Poulsen, P., H.H. Smedegaard, J. Roed, and E. Korsgaard. 1994. Equine hoof function investigated by pressure transducers inside the hoof and accelerometers mounted on the first phalanx. *Equine Veterinary Journal* 26, no. 5: 362-366.

Hood, D.M., N.W. Burt, S.J. Baker, and I.P. Wagner. 1997. Effects of Ground Surface on Solar Load Distribution. *AAEP Proceedings* 43: 360-362.

Leach, Doug. 1982. The Structure and Function of the Equine Hoof. *American Farriers Journal* : 11-15.

Lungwitz, A. 1891. The Changes in the Form of the Horse's Hoof Under the Action of the Body-Weight. *Journal of Comparative Pathology and Therapeutics* 4, no. 3: 191–211.

Page, Barbara. 2001. Evaluating the position of the coffin bone relative to the hoof capsule. *Journal of Equine Veterinary Science* 21, no. 6: 297.

Page, Barbara T. and Tracey L. Hagen. 2002. Breakover of the hoof and its effect on structures and forces within the foot. *Journal of Equine Veterinary Science* 2, no. 6: 258-263.

Chapter 6
Laminitis

Curtis, Simon, Dave W. Ferguson, Randy Luikart, and Gene Ovnicek. 1999. Trimming and Shoeing the Chronically Affected Horse. *Veterinary Clinics of North America: Equine Practice* 15, no. 2: 463-480.

Harman, Joyce and Madalyn Ward. 2000. Laminitis Treatment: A Natural Medicine Perspective. *Hoofcare and Lameness Journal of Equine Foot Science*, no. 73.

Hood, David M. 1999. Laminitis as a Systemic Disease. *Veterinary Clinics of North America: Equine Practice* 15, no. 2: 481-494.

Hood, David M., Max S. Amoss, and Deborah A. Grosenbaugh. 1990. Equine Laminitis: A Potential Model of Raynaud's Phenomenon. *Angiology Journal of Vascular Diseases* 41, no. 4: 270-277.

Linford, Robert, Timothy R. O'Brien, and Donald R. Trout. 1993. Qualitative and morphometric radiographic findings in the distal phalanx and digital soft tissues of sound Thoroughbred racehorses. *American Journal of Veterinary Research* 54, no. 1: 38-51.

Mungall, Bruce A., Myat Kyaw-Tanner, and Christopher C. Pollitt. 2001. In vitro evidence for a bacterial pathogenesis of equine laminitis. *Veterinary Microbiology* 79: 209-223.

Page, B.T., R.M. Bowker, G. Ovnicek, and T. Hagen. 1999. How to mark the hoof for radiography. *Proceedings of the 45th Annual Convention of the American Association of Equine Practitioners* 45.

Pollitt, Christopher C. 2003. Equine Laminitis. In *Proceedings of the 49th Annual Convention of the American Association of Equine Practitioners*, 49:103-115. New Orleans, Louisiana: AAEP.

Redden, Ric R. 2003. Clinical and Radiographic Examination of the Equine Foot. In *Proceedings of the 49th Annual Convention of the American Association of Equine Practitioners*, 49:169-185. New Orleans: AAEP.

Wagner, Ilka P., Christine A. Rees, Robert W. Dunstan, Kelly M. Credille, and David M. Hood. 2003. Evaluation of systemic immunologic hyperreactivity after intradermal testing in horses with chronic laminitis. *American Journal of Veterinary Research* 64, no. 3: 279-283.

Navicular

Bowker, Robert M., Patrick J. Atkinson, Theresa S. Atkinson, and Roger C. Haut. 2001. Effect of contact stress in bones of the distal interphalangeal joint on microscopic changes in articular cartilage and ligaments. *American Journal of Veterinary Research* 62, no. 3: 414-424.

Bowker, Robert M., Kimberly K. Van Wulfen, Susan E. Springer, and Keith E. Linder. 1998. Functional anatomy of the cartilage of the distal phalanx and digital cushion in the equine foot and a hemodynamic flow hypothesis of energy dissipation. *American Journal of Veterinary Research* 59, no. 8: 961-968.

Leach, D.H. 1993. Treatment and pathogenesis of navicular disease ('syndrome') in horses. *Equine Veterinary Journal* 25, no. 6: 477-481.

Viitanen, M.J., A.M. Wilson, H.P. McGuigan, K.D. Rogers, and S.A. May. 2003. Effect of foot balance on the intra-articular pressure in the distal interphalangeal joint *in vitro*. *Equine Veterinary Journal* 35, no. 2: 184-189.

Willemen, M.A., H.H.C.M. Savelberg, and A. Barneveld. 1999. The effect of orthopaedic shoeing on the force exerted by the deep digital flexor tendon on the navicular bone in horses. *Equine Veterinary Journal* 33, no. 1: 25-30.

Wilson, A.M., M.P. McGuigan, L. Fouracre, and L. MacMahon. 2001. The force and contact stress on the navicular bone during trot locomotion in sound horses and horses with navicular disease. *Equine Veterinary Journal* 33, no. 2: 159-165.

Note: A complete bibliography is available at www.lancasterequine.com

Photography and Art Credits

Page 2	John Miller/Spectrum Photography
Fig 2.9	Kara Nichole Corps
Fig 2.11	Kara Nichole Corps
Fig 3.13	John Miller/Spectrum Photography
Fig 4.5	Kara Nichole Corps
Fig 5.4	John Miller/Spectrum Photography
Fig 5.6	John Miller/Spectrum Photography
Fig 5.8	Andrea Flaks
Fig 6.13	Robert Bowker
Fig 6.14	Robert Bowker
Fig 6.15	Kara Nichole Corps
Fig 8.1	Star Ridge Publishing
Fig 8.2	Mona Kay
Fig 8.3	Jim Stoner Photography
Fig 8.4	Jamie Saycocie
Fig 8.5	Springer
Fig 8.6	Kandi Schuman
Fig 8.7	Creative Photography
Fig 8.8	Maria Villenevue
Fig 8.9	Darolyn Butler-Dial
Fig 8.11	Larry Larson
Fig 8.12	Deb Harper
Fig 8.13	Deb Harper
Fig 8.14	Star Ridge Publishing
Fig 8.15	Creative Photography
Fig 8.16	Sue Greenall
Fig 8.17	Phebe Peterson
Fig 8.18	Rick Lancaster
Fig 8.19	Sheila McAttee
Fig 8.20	www.tribeequus.com
Fig 8.21	www.tribeequus.com
Fig 8.22	Kirt Lander

Index

A
Anatomy 7
   Anatomical planes 7

B
Balance 37
   Medio-Lateral Symmetry 42
   Toe to Heel 40
Bowker, Robert 15, 88, 90
Breakover 27
Butler, Doug 41, 50, 66

C
Coffin Bone 9
Contraction 60

D
Digital Cushion 17, 48, 89
Duckett, Dave 39
   Duckett's Bridge 40
   Duckett's Dot 40

E
Expansion (see Hoof deformation)
Extensor Process 8, 51

F
Four-Point trim 52
Frog 12, 16, 33

G
Growth Rings 31, 84

H
Hairline 29, 44, 80, 94
Heel Length 25
Heel Pain 86, 89, 90, 91
Holistic Hoof Care 1, 57, 113
Hood, David 53, 76
Hoof-Pastern Axis 25, 29, 44, 52, 68, 82, 89
Hoof Deformation 46, 76
Hoof Moisture 32
Hoof Shape 27
Hoof Wall 25, 29, 31, 42

L
Laminae 15
Laminitis 4, 36, 45, 57, 73, 74, 80
   Clinical Signs 76, 81, 83, 85
   Diagnosis 84
   Treatment 74, 77, 84
Lateral Cartilage 17, 30, 54, 88, 89

N
Natural Balance 13, 52, 53, 117
Navicular Bone 10, 41, 52, 54, 85, 87
Navicular Syndrome 73, 85, 90

O
Ovnicek, Gene 13, 41, 51, 84, 117

P
P3 9, 44, 48, 50, 74, 81, 82
Palmar Process 9, 10, 17, 30, 48
Pastern Bone 8, 11, 82, 90
Pollitt, Chris 74
Proximal 8, 17

R
Record Keeping 97
Redden, Ric 52, 80
Rotation 82
   Capsular 81, 82
   Phalangeal 82, 88

S
Sesamoid Bone 11
Shoes
   Clips 67
   Nails 64, 65, 69
   Shape 65
   Size 66
Solar Surface Proportions 32, 41
Sole 13, 15, 34, 54, 81

T
Toe Length 25, 40

W
White Line 14, 27, 36, 52, 54, 62, 70

X
X-rays 80, 85

Acknowledgements

I extend a heartfelt thanks to the following people, all of whom have contributed in some way to my professional development and the writing of this book. Mistakes and misinterpretations are my own. Thank you:

To my publishers, Amy Snow and Nancy Zidonis, for their faith in this project from its beginnings in a hoof care seminar they attended years ago, and for their pioneering work in holistic therapies and education for animal care providers.

To my shoeing school instructor, Mark Russell, for giving me a sound start in the basics. The first day I trimmed a hoof I said to Mark, "I'm scared." And he said, "You should be scared! That's a live foot you are taking sharp tools to. The horse has no choice but to walk on those feet when you're finished. Don't ever forget that."

To farriers Dave Duckett, Henry Heymering, and Gene Ovnicek for their contributions to farrier education and their leadership in hoof care today.

To Jaime Jackson, for his wild horse work, his belief in the horse owning public, and his leadership in the natural hoof care movement.

To researcher Bob Bowker, for his "out of the box" thinking and for his patience while I fumbled around his lab trying to learn histology. For his steadfast determination to discover the world inside the horse's hoof.

To my clients and friends in the horse world, from Vermont to Colorado to Wyoming to Michigan, too numerous to list here. You know who you are, and what you are to me.

To farrier and equine veterinarian Tia Nelson, for her unflagging support of my struggle as "just a farrier" to stick with it through vet school.

To my parents, Margaret and Tony Simons, for always believing in me.

To Fran Jurga, for steering me in the right direction every step of way since the day I finished shoeing school. For all she has done for horses. For her tireless dedication to the hoof care world. For promoting hoof and horse sense from a "feet first" perspective. For being the center of everything hoof.

To my husband, John, for more than words can capture.

To my lifelong best friend, my sister Rachel, for every little thing.

About the Author

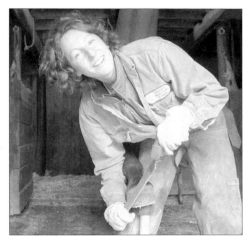

Farrier Lisa S. Lancaster has been trimming and shoeing horses since 1998. Her practice emphasizes education for horse owners in holistic hoof care. She trained at the Colorado School of Trades, and is a member of the American Farrier's Association.

Lisa grew up in New England and learned horsemanship as a member of the 4-H and US Pony Club organizations. For over 30 years she has been riding, training and competing horses, participating in various disciplines including dressage, distance riding, and combined driving.

Lisa acquired her PhD from the University of Denver and at the time of publication of this book was completing her doctor of veterinary medicine. Concurrently, she was earning a Masters degree researching microanatomy of the horse's hoof.

Lisa lives in Colorado with her husband, John.

ORDER FORM

EQUINE

NEW The Sound Hoof: Horse Health From the Ground Up $26.95
Equine Acupressure: A Working Manual. $29.95
Equine Meridian Chart. 12 x 18 color, laminated chart. $16.00
Equine Stretch Poster. 12 x 18 laminated poster. $16.00

Five-Element Meridian Chart Set. Includes 4 – 12 x 18 color, laminated charts of meridian system: 14 Major Meridians, Accumulation, Alarm Association, Command, Connecting, Source and Ting Points. Plus Five-Element Theory chart. $53.50

INTRODUCING Equine Acupressure: A Training Video - A 50 minute hands-on training & demonstration video. Details Opening, Point Work and Closing Techniques & specific point location and point combinations. $39.95

FELINE

Acu-Cat: A Guide to Feline Acupressure. $23.95
Feline Meridian Chart. 12 x 18 color, laminated chart. $16.00

CANINE

The Well Connected Dog: A Guide to Canine Acupressure. $25.95
Canine Meridian Chart. 12 x 18 color, laminated chart. $16.00

Name_____ Phone_____

Street/POB _____

City/State/Zip_____

Email _____

ITEM	DESCRIPTION	QTY	UNIT PRICE	TOTAL AMT
SHP & HNDLG			Sub-Total	
Canada $9.00			CO 3.8%	
1-3 bks / charts $6			S&H	
3-6 bks/chrts $9			TOTAL	

PAYMENT: MC/VISA #   EXP DATE:

TO ORDER: Call: 1-888-841-7211

e-mail tallgrasspub@earthlink.net or acupressure4all@earthlink.net

SEND TO: Tallgrass Publishers LLC, 4559 Red Rock Dr., Larkspur, CO 80118

Website: www.tallgrasspublishers.com **or** www.animalacupressure.com